Auto-Immune Heresy
A Memoir
Laure Marin de la Vallée

Hemochrome Press

First Edition © 2024, Laure Marin de la Vallée

All rights reserved. No portion of this book may be reproduced in any form without written permission from the publisher or author, except for brief quotations in critical articles or reviews, and to share it with your friends.

Self-published in 2024

Email: contact@laure.love

Visit www.laure.love

Front cover art by Meagan Chaput

All other illustrations and photographs by the author

Paperback ISBN: 978-1-7382769-0-5

Ebook ISBN: 978-1-7382769-1-2

À Maman
To the bees
To the ghosts
L'chaim!

47. ASSEZ! Nous nous mutinons. Nous fermons l'usine où nous fabriquons le sang, où nous dosons les globules rouges et les globules blancs.
                              Louky Bersianik, L'Euguélionne

*The things of this world
exist, they are;
you cannot refuse them.*
                              U.K Leguin rendering Lao Tze

Contents

Preface	IX
1. Questions For A Blood Doctor	1
General Guidelines	8
A Chameleon Ethic	14
Total Hyphema and Childhood Glaucoma	20
Dreamt	25
I Reviewed This Nice Boy	32
Receiving A Dose	36
B-12 Adventures	40
A Visit To The Blood Doctor	43
Becoming Sick, Becoming Trans	46
Photophobia and Blind Gain	49
2. Sickness As A Way Of Life	55
You Matter	62
Digressions	67
38.5 degrees centigrade	69
Sharing Air	79

A Little Golden Cat	82
Sympathie Sanguine	85
Longing for Heat	91
The Oncology Ward In The Sky	93
3. Patience	97
Taking Back My Body	106
Communion	110
Regressing Moves Forward	114
Reading Phaedrus	126
Vein To Vial	128
Waiting	148
Sickness in Limbo	167
A Spring Spent Nannying	174
4. Surrender	179
Auto-Immune Manifesto	180
New Asceticism	181
Omnia mutantur	185
All Things Change	198
Smaller, still	204
At the end // À Suivre	206
Selected Bibliography	209
About Laure	211

Preface

My body is auto-immune.
That means I must learn how it responds to the world.

I used to trust doctoring,
the way a child trusts warm-hearted adults.
It took 20 years to learn
that I know my body better than anyone else.

I am not a marble statue.
I am sick of the metal leeches
which have taken a hundred hundred measures of blood
only to declare it pathological.

This is a story I've been preparing to tell.
These texts result from 8 years of writing.
They take as material over two decades of my own life,
my thoughts and feelings about the world into which I am launched.

I make no claims about the ultimate truth of what I say.
The stories here are biography, flights of fancy, dream,
memory, recollection, conversation, fabulation, speculation.
If I were selling to French literary publishers
I would call this an auto-fiction.
If I were selling to alternative scholarly presses
I would call it auto-theory.
As it stands, the small press distributing this book needed no sales pitch.
I write, so that these words may go out to all interested parties.
May what needs to be heard be heard.

Blood is sticky.
It is fundamental to our lives, and too often ignored.
Here, it takes center stage, its cup runneth over.

For whom is life not a sickness?
Leaving the house laden with burdens,
illness is never long forgotten.

Beginning the telling fills me with trepidation. My heart knows that reliving these events won't be easy for me, and would almost rather keep silent, not bother sharing. With the encouragement and support of many friends, I take a step forward, and begin.

It was 2001, high summer near the Salish Sea of Turtle Island's Pacific northwest. So-called Vancouver, British Columbia. I was 5 years old. Life was a series of forest adventures, pre-school friendships, and creative curiosities held warmly by my single mother's devotion to raising a child alone in her 40s. Being from colonized Gespe'gewa'gi on the opposite ocean's shore, she had made home in Vancouver during an early adulthood spent traveling the world, fuelled by pure curiosity. She was ready to have a child. Though her lover decided he couldn't be a father, she chose to become a mother.

Surrounded by friends, she brought me into a world full of infinite possibility. She recounted myths and fed my love of story. We laughed to the point of tears as she read me kid-friendly renditions of the judeo-christian tradition; we imagined a world of justice and love, as she nourished us both with tales of equality and ecology--new myths for a changing planet.

I remember the story of a young princess, dark of skin, who ventures into the enchanted forest. She gets lost, lost in her fear of the woods, fear she received from her father. So the guardians of the ancient groves, a dragon and a unicorn, show her how the forest is a place of beauty. When the princess returns home, she shows her father, and he recognizes his daughter's wisdom. He changes his ways. He stops destroying the forest.

I grew up feeling like the forest held all the world's magic, all its wisdom. I knew this to be the truth. My home was an environment in which this ecstatic curiosity and passion for the world, its arts, its stories, could flourish.

There are many things my mother did not know, but she transmitted the pieces that mattered. She underscored that in all the stories, and in all our relations, the uniting, healing force, the bridge across enmity and the conflictual sense of separateness, is love. As she shared the stories of Adam, Abraham, Moses, she did not have the biting historical comparative-mythology political-philosophy gender-studies critique I would develop two decades later, when I went back to the scripture. Her love of God was as simple and as pure as her love of a child she named Matthieu-Xavier Marin. After the apostle, whose name she made a point of telling me means "gift from god"--and her own father, François-Xavier, a Gaspésien through-and-through, a heavy machinery mechanic whose career was spent in Murdochville's copper mine.

It was 2001, and I was 5 years old. Summer was coming to a head, the temperate rainforest soaked up the sun's rays. My days were filled with play, with harmless games. One of those days, my friend and I were brought to a seaside market gift-shop. My memories of Vancouver's markets are fond. I remember the smell of salt on the air, the smoked salmon, the honey candies. I remember the seagulls arguing over the leftover fries from the fish n' chips stalls. I can still taste the mango sorbet.

This story begins by accident.

"We can't treat this,"
told us the walk-in clinic attendant,
"go to the hospital."

And so we did.

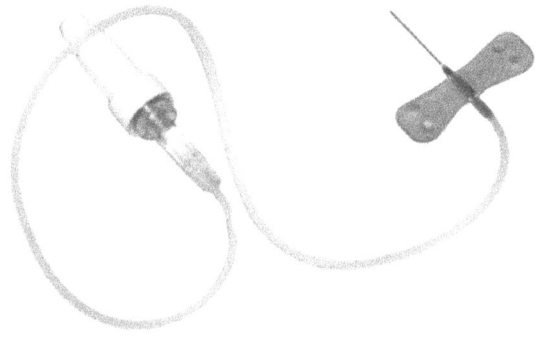

Questions For A Blood Doctor

DATE	PLATELET	PREDNISONE	OTHER Rx	
10-Aug-01	<5		IVIG	
11-Aug-01	<5		IVIG	
12-Aug-01	<5			
13-Aug	7			Bone marrow
14-Aug-01	<5			
15-Aug-01	<5	2mg/kg		
16-Aug-01	11	2mg/kg		
17-Aug-01	16	2mg/kg		
18-Aug-01	14	2mg/kg		
19-Aug-01	14	2mg/kg		
20-Aug-01	27	2mg/kg		
23-Aug-01	8	2mg/kg		
27-Aug-01	10	2mg/kg	Anti-D IgG	
31-Aug-01	7	2mg/kg		
04-Sep-01	<5	2mg/kg		
07-Sep-01	6	2mg/kg		
13-Sep-01	6	2mg/kg	Dexamethasone	
18-Sep-01	17	wean		
21-Sep-01	7	wean		
25-Sep-01	<5	wean		
28-Sep-01	151	wean		
29-Sep-01	140	wean		
30-Sep-01	168	wean		
01-Oct-01	207	wean		
05-Oct-01	279	wean		
11-Oct-01	62	wean		
12-Oct-01	63	wean		
17-Oct-01	71	off		
24-Oct-01	31	off		
31-Oct-01	33	off		
07-Nov-01	28	off		
13-Nov-01	26	off		
21-Nov-01	18	off		
27-Nov-01	18			
04-Dec-01	12			
12-Dec-01	102		Dexamethasone	
18-Dec-01	29			
24-Dec-01	14			
31-Dec-01	23			
08-Jan-02	16		Dexamethasone	
15-Jan-02	95			
29-Jan-01	19			
05-Feb-02	27			
12-Feb-02	15			
19-Feb-02	8		Dexamethasone	
26-Feb-02	173			
12-Mar-02	32			
20-Mar-02	34			
26-Mar-02	10		Dexamethasone	
02-Apr-02	176			
14-May-02	44			

THERE ONCE WAS A boy.
No, that's not quite the word.

There once was a pussy willow lounging in the reeds
with nowhere to call but home
when the days ran out of tune
like the great-grandfather's marine band harp,
rusty with a half-century's dis-use,
still sounded crystal clear carrion call
on the neatly tended forest path
wide, and cleared by hundreds of feet each day.

At a glance no wilds remain here.
So she buys a new harmonica
the same model, tuned to G
It don't sound the same.
Within a day the 3rd reed broke
(won't play on the inhale)
but she don't give up because
the harp's got something to teach
her diaphragm about waking up to use,
what's more it seems like a neat campfire
side doodad to pluck from a pocket
when the time is ripe.

Always thinking about how to gather
around the fire, now that I've had
a taste again. Israel was
the man's name, we spoke for hours
letting our tongues weave new
old folklore for the current apocalypse,
stories tuned to the beat of the tongue-drum
with only beauty and time on our hands,
though liquor too in his case,
not mine.

How could I keep doing this,
if I had to to do it forever?
I remember to pray. Do it over again.
Repeat, reread, rewrite.
Bow, and remember reverence.
Again, again. Practice { }
Don't presume to know what the day holds.

If it were simple maybe I'd need not repeat myself
and repeat myself. If it were complex
maybe saying it once would suffice
to anchor the pattern.
If there were a perceptible logic
then simplicity would occur.
But, no, logic breeds the complicated
the reasoned, the interminable excuses.
Simple is the path to health, one breath at a time,
one refusal after another.
I still don't want your cure, Doctor.
I still think you've got it wrong, Doctor.
Let's grab a drink and laugh about it.
Let's get down to the business
of coming to terms with impending,
ongoing collapse. What's the matter, doctor?
Was that a threat?

You tell me that if so-called alternative treatment fails,
I may not be get back on these meds?
You say that the adjudicators are only human,
and so their reasoning may be:
"Oh, well, if they wanted to go try natural medicine,
why should we re-approve this expense?"
Doctor, I am confused.
Why is it that my desire to seek other care
may later be punished?
Humans, you say?
No, I am not so sure the impulse driving bureaucrats
is a human agenda.

Tell me doctor,
how quickly do we fall through the cracks once our dissent is known
to the legalese-fluent contract-dependent policy-breathing sort?
How little does it take for us to get blacklisted?
One misstep, or two?
I say, Doctor, your thinly veiled threat sits with me.
You wish me luck and pawn me off
to a specialist nearer-by
as if you haematologists treat bodies, not numbers.
You make me sick, don't make me laugh.
No, I would not rather be healthy, no thanks to you.

Here, take some clonazepam, you'll
quickly feel better, then worse, then
take another, and soon enough
the numbness will forestall all
capacity for worry. Come on, let's
go for a joyride. Oil's pricey, sure,
but on your specialists' salary?
Indulge a bit. Get a friend
to write that prescription for you
sure beats sitting in a waiting room,
waiting to see the psych,
knowing a fabulous act
is about to be put on display.
Depression's a game we play
on stage, hide behind a mask
of lights and pills, and whisper
into the lonely pillow at
the end of the 80 hour work week.

Orientation's finding your way,
feeling at home goes unnoticed
until lost, disorientation results. Lost,
unable to navigate and find my way.

I do not know how I'm supposed to relate to my body.
It is mine with which to do as I please,
to care for and mutilate and experiment with.
Yet I am at a loss, learning
to navigate tides of being.

A sick body is a magical labyrinth,
full of shifting corridors and dead ends.
To orient myself in this world, I rely on this labyrinth.
I trust that it will guide me where we need to go.
I am not the architect, only a passenger.

A life lived through medicine is an incomplete form of existence,
one which foregoes so much agency,
which must trust in the expertise
of sometimes personally disagreeable individuals.

The architects thus far have been
those whose signatures prescribe my physiology.
Being diagnosed and treated is akin
to a long game of pin the tale on the donkey,
where the patient is both blindfolded and the donkey itself.

Who better to undertake the journey through the depths?
A glacier mountain ridge-line crawling single-file
with pilgrims seeking a detour and a view.
Embraced by the cold morning.
Do go carefully, ye who seek alleged salvation.
Are we not living beings?
What greater opportunity for joy?
The inner grammar of sensation resounds
with gnosis if ye only tune to listen.

There is much embedded in the texts
which drive my striving, but perhaps the answers
better yet, the questions
reside merely in the flesh borne of mother's womb.

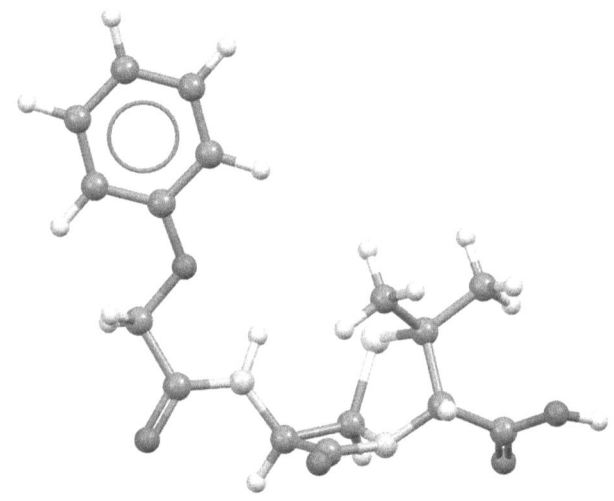

General Guidelines

I AM LOOKING AT an image.
A single page photocopy of an informational handout.
It is titled "General Guidelines for the Management of a Child with ITP"
In all likelihood, it was among the first documents that Maman received from healthcare professionals after my diagnosis in 2001, and it appears to be directed at schoolteachers. It's a little bit outdated. Most notably, ITP is now called 'Immune Thrombocytopenia' rather than 'Idiopathic Thrombocytopenic Purpura', and there are more treatment options than two decades ago.
Writing in 2019, I have had an ITP diagnosis for 18 years.
Research from 2018 estimates that immune thrombocytopenia is found in 8.8 out of 100'000 children.
The same research also finds that in 25% of ITP cases, the condition becomes chronic, persistent: it does not simply go away. New diagnosis: Chronic Immune Thrombocytopenia, found in 2.2 out of 100'000 children.

I'm struck by a particular choice of words in the pamphlet:
"benign disease."
Medical conditions are called benign to suggest they are not dangerous or serious. Benign can also mean kind, or kindly. I am one of the few whose so-called benign disease turned into the chronic form.
As if auto-immunity were ever benign.

                              In the first months of treatment
                    from August 10 2001 to May 14 2002,
                                    I received steroids,
                  intravenous immunoglobulin (IVIG),
                                          Prednisone,
                                        51 blood tests,
                  Rho(D) immune globulin (RhIG)
                                     Dexamethasone,
                             a bone marrow biopsy,
                       and had my spleen removed.

                          After which, I took penicillin
                         (NOVO-PEN-VK 500 300MG)
                                                 daily
                                      for a decade.
                 (wikipedia: Phenoxymethylpenicillin)

Treatment is still only ever palliative,
meaning that doctors manage symptoms
but do not seek a cure.
My ITP has always been around,
and anytime my immune system is activated,
it seeks out and destroys my platelets.
Platelets are an essential clotting factor.

Auto-immunity is endlessly alienating and confusing. As a kid, I understood logically that I 'was sick' and might someday 'get better' but was wholly unequipped to deal with the emotional and psychological repercussions of living with a body that may or may not be bleeding at all times.

Think of it this way: my body is a black box and my veins are Schrödinger's cat.

The handout also has a very limited definition of "life style" but does capture the restrictions imposed upon the child. Immunosuppressed to avoid self-destruction, disallowed bodily contact sports to avoid potential external dangers. I was an isolated kid, but I don't mean to sound down about it all. I turned out alright, but yeah, it sucked at the time.

This document provided general information and guidelines for managing me, the child with ITP. It was intended for adults to have at least a vague sense of what was Wrong™ with me and adjust their treatment accordingly. As far as I recall, I never got a handout. Or counselling, until I sought it out myself 15 years down the line.

It is my intention in this book to vulgarize and translate my experience of illness in such a way as to be informative and engaging. I am telling you a story. I want to share what I've been through, in the hope that my words will resonate with others. I am not a doctor, I was a patient.

In attempting to show the research I do, I may get things wrong.

I ask that you forgive such errors as you notice,

and engage in a dialogue with me.

Thanks to Maman's record keeping, I have a filing cabinet of my medical transcripts, letters, general information and the like, which covers most of my childhood post-diagnosis.

This is where I begin to disentangle it. I am setting out on an archaeological dig of the medical knowledge that was produced about me.

2019-09-27

From The Hospital On The Day Of The Climate March

At the oncology-haematology clinic,
   the wait time was only about 8 minutes.
The CHUM's 14th floor waiting room's got a wall of windows
into the azure and the river.

Portable FM feeds my earbuds live coverage of the day's main event.
A guest-host panders to us all, repeating that everyone has limits they must
   face, that we must all contend with ourselves and do what we can within
   our communities, that one of the great projects for anyone who is alive
   right now is to try being as human as possible within dehumanizing
   systems.
Blood test took all of 30 seconds.
Routine.

Next, 12 floors down, tucked away above the main entrance, lounges
   Gastroenterology, where the blue room has no windows. I checked in
   early, 10:12, hopeful I'd have some energy left over to march.
Finally, noon, was not greeted by a doctor.
The desk clerk asks me: "Can you come back next week?"
Due to a system error, the MD wasn't notified of my arrival.
So the time had passed. She couldn't see me.
Next week? Huh. Ok.

At least I have the institutional note from the day of the climate march.
I stayed tuned in to radio coverage as I left the hospital, north then west,
   arrived at Saint-Laurent metro, and watched the crowd.
Heard it and and its cries many minutes before
eyes glimpsed details of its millipede limbs over groaning asphalt.
Contingents of friends singers dancers rolling, celebrating,

all blended into the marching worm wafting
despair
and jouissance.
Sticking from the ground were red and yellow metal acoustic tubes,
distorting and delaying the cheers and chants.
There, in the streets, bidding farewell to the earth,
were so many of us, it is haunting.

There's bitter irony I have not yet resolved
in facing obstacles to action imposed by a body
having only just the energy to survive and remain calm.
Doubtless, many of the people attending
to waiting rooms that day wished to be demonstrating instead.
We too wanted to feel a part of a seething mass.
Instead, we patiently sat in chairs, awaiting expert examination,
hoping our bodily prognosis is better than that of this earth.

A slow gunmetal ooze creeps like magma
but does not glow or emit its warmth.
Pressure mounts in my chest a clarion-call
noiseless signal that life remains, pains and all.
Awake to the body's below-all-the-dust and roses there
exists a self which, shaped by the world, surpasses it.
Transcendent to the last day. A self a precious few find
thanks to the forces of circumstance.
Anchored and buoyed along the path I am
soothed in my frenzied preparations by reminders to slow down.
My lifeline in a frenzy of deadlines is continuous
awareness that the worlds within me sap the world.
Each new attempt is faced with greater knowledge
and skill. Baggage is a dirty word, but with it comes
a survival guide. Tools of the mind and soul
to equip and take on life's trials.

AUTO-IMMUNE HERESY

I hear within myself: You are not doing enough.
That voice may always be there.
There is no other way to exist in a world that is ending
but community support.
Nothing to be done except mutual aid,
the creation of spaces for grief and joy.
So what now?
Perhaps calm is a coping mechanism,
because to lose calm is to fall far, deep, lost.
unsustainable emotions when there are bills due on the 1st.
I just try to get enough sleep.

A Chameleon Ethic

PARALLELS CAN BE DRAWN between trans experience and chronic illness,
   but making up a list won't get at the truth of it.
So many knots in my chest leave me uneasy.
I try to sit with them and feel them out
but untangling roots is often more than I can do alone.
I try not to retreat into numbness, with its familiar haze.
When I let myself numb to life, I lose the magic that is: feeling.
Emotions are exhausting, but at least they are true.

I've been sick so long that I forget what an effect illness has on life.
Let me be clear, when I say illness, I don't mean an occasional cold/flu.
I mean long-term, recurring, full of unknowns
no matter how many test results pile up in a file.
When I speak of illness I mean the ever-present sense of bodily doubt,
of not knowing whether it will ever be possible to trust my body.
Radical Left politics of anti-ableism would have me accept my illness.
My leanings toward a zen worldview would as well.
But how can I possibly be equanimous?
My mind is riddled with self-judgement at my body's
inability to keep up, ever after all the years.

I figure maybe I'll Get Better.
Better implying an inherent lack in sick bodies.
Better positing that sick bodies are
    unable to conduct themselves in valuable ways.
Better stating that illness is morally
    inferior to health, and so it is for its bearer.
Better implying that a body's worth is
    determined by their ability to generate surplus value.
Better making clear that value only exists
    outside the cycle of chronic illness.
Better saying that there is no value
    in the process of perpetual healing.
Better affirming
    "you'd be happier if you were healthy."
Better reminding us that sick bodies are
    to be pitied for their state of being.
What is truly meant when stating Get Better is:
    get back to work.

I say I don't "function properly", as if my body were a machine
"Keep up", as if I'm running a footrace and my body is dragging down the
    team.
The truth is that my body can not and will not
ever operate at any rhythm or capacity other than its own.

I've burned out every other year since turning 18,
and each time I get back on my feet after some period of unproductivity,
I wonder how to better make Being Productive a sustainable endeavour.

My thinking is inherently flawed,
and is the result of capital's insidious grasp over my mind.
Inherently flawed, because I am thinking about my body as the problem,
as a puzzle to be cracked.

If I only eat right, exercise, meditate, don't drink, take my meds, sleep 9
    hours a night…
THEN I'll Be Better enough to exist frictionlessly.
Injunctions such as Be Well turn the well-meaning speaker
into a prophet upholding morality, that false virtue of health.

They tell you to be well
and parrot the priestly call to piety.
How many patients internalize a narrative
of illness as punishment for some wrongdoing?
The end of that story is cure through repentance.

My desire to get better is only rivalled by my rage at the inescapability of the system
that perpetually makes unsustainable demands of all bodies,
sick or otherwise, human or otherwise, living or otherwise.

I try to develop all the right habits and I still find myself in crisis. I scramble for self-preservation only to find that everyone else is sinking too. No amount of internalized wellness rhetoric changes that my body is prone to random bouts of self-destruction, that the structures that guide labour and consumption as they exist today make no affordances for predictably unpredictable health. I work 40 hours a week because it seems like the thing to do. Because is seems like having a steady paycheck that lets me do more than just survive may be worth it.

But what is it really worth?
Is it worth my mental health to take any job with a salary and dissociate 8 hours a day?
Is it worth the energy commitment, not having enough left over
to see my loved ones even kind of regularly?
Is it worth the feelings of isolation that comes with being
a closeted trans in a Progressive™ office environment?
The kind of place that has social-inclusion policies in place, though their efficacy is doubtful at best.
Is it worth creating friction in the system in order to Live My Identity?
Or would my identity be better lived elsewhere?

As I write this, I'm about to embark on an overnight laxative journey
in order to adequately prepare myself for a colonoscopy
scheduled tomorrow morning.
A look inside my bowels to check if I'm bleeding.
They're looking for the cause of my anemia,
as if ITP wasn't enough of an answer.
I suppose that Medically Speaking, it isn't.
It had been over 2 years since I last visited with the gastroenterologist, and
 our meeting lasted less than 10 minutes. Dr. Guts looked at my numbers
 and evinced confusion:
"Your iron is still low," she said,
"and... your platelets jumped from 19 to 427 last April."
"Yes," I confirmed, "I rested that month."
"Your platelets shot that high because you...rested?"
"Yes, that's what I said."
My platelets were low when I checked into the ER in late that one night
 in March 2019 due to high fever. I spent the night sitting under fluorescents in a half-lotus, listening, taking in the noise. My regular blood
 doctor was the attendant haematologist, and he upped my regular meds
 when he got around to my hallway-bound cot at 7am the next morning.
 So in April the meds I was taking everyday were doing their thing,
 too. My haematologist and I have a decent working relationship. He's
 followed my case since I was 19, he knows what my body's up to.
Dr. Guts, the gastroenterologist, I saw for the first time in 2017 when by
 her careful hand tubes with cameras insinuated through me to check
 whether some part of my large intestine or bowels was bleeding. They
 were not. The experience was deeply troubling. Perhaps some of you
 have been through this procedure: Drugged to near-total dissociation
 with fentanyl, I was out cold for the majority of the invasion. I had
 a single moment of lucidity. My oesophagus was occupied by plastic,
 my intestine shifting uneasily to accommodate the probe. I was aware
 of movement inside me. Not alarmed, not in pain, only aware. My
 stomach, distended in odd ways, occupied my attention. I did not see.
 I knew what was happening, what I had agreed to. I waited, patiently,
 comatose. They found my insides to be positively normal.

Dr. Guts: "After the procedure in 2017,
I prescribed you iron supplement pills."
"Yes," I acquiesced, "they stopped working."
"They worked for a while," she points out astutely.
Research has found that oral iron supplement treatments generally take 6-8 months to fix the problem and restore the body's iron levels. Two years after the little red pills, my iron levels have generally remained quite low, my iron-deficiency anaemia without a clear fix. From April to May 2019, I received iron intravenously.
That almost did the trick.
Since the original procedure in 2017, I have twice received undiscussed and unexpected summons for another gastroscopy-endoscopy, in spite of my doctor confirming that the original examination and accompanying biopsies yielded no results. Part of me thinks Dr. Guts just really enjoys performing this particular test.
Until now, I have refused to undergo the procedure again. We've discussed other options, so I remain confused as to why that procedure was requisitioned again. Yet here we are, December 2019, and tomorrow they're checking.
I agreed to this. I'm afraid of the consequences of not following medical orders. I spend a lot of my time concerned with the personal/political consequences of ingesting such and such food or media product. I feel so porous, affected by everything I consume, medicine included. When it comes to medical orders, I follow them critically. That is to say, I follow them. I do not presume to know how to balance my body's chemical load better than my MDs. I feel how the variety of medications affect me, but currently lack knowledge about their biological functioning or the targets we are trying to reach. Even though I doubt anything will come
from this test or the next, I agree.
Because I know this:
a normal amount of blood platelets is 150'000-300'000 per microliter of blood,
and my counts in 2019, after 18 blood tests, have been between 9000 and 427'000.

When I do what I'm told, they stabilize;
when I forget to take meds, omit to fill a prescription,
or otherwise live life counter to medical recommendations,
they plummet.

So, each evening,
I take a small orange pill marked 50mg,
and a white one marked 25mg of the same.

Having chronic illness means giving up a degree of agency that many
    people take for granted.
I don't have control over what doctors decide is necessary for my body.
That's distressing, but I still have trust that the public-system
specialists who examine me have my Health (nebulous concept) in mind.
The same cannot be said for many other ways
in which bodily autonomy is taken from individuals.
The medical violence I experience as a byproduct of treatment is of the
    softest sort.
I'm working class, but I haven't fallen through the cracks.
I am, for all intents and purposes in the medical system, a man.
I am not out there seeking hormone replacement therapy.
And why not?
I barely have the energy to make it through my weeks
I am not about to compound that
with the social burden of coming out
to everyone everywhere all the time.
I don't have the courage.

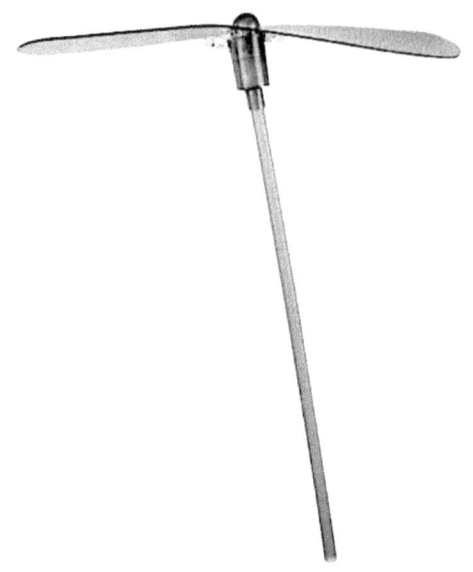

Total Hyphema and Childhood Glaucoma

I AM LOOKING AT a letter that was faxed from my then-ophthalmologist (eye doctor) in Vancouver to my soon-ophthalmologist in Ottawa.

Right before I was diagnosed with Immune Thrombocytopenia, I was playing by myself while I waited for Maman to finish meeting with my Waldorf school kindergarten teacher. I had just been given back a toy that was confiscated and I was very excited to resume playing with it.

As fate would have it, the spinning toy turned on me and flew at my right eye, causing permanent damage.

It was a red day.
Red as to stain my vision.
Red with weep, sorrow.
Red with pain, confusion.
Red like the couches and the carpets
 in the first clinic my mother brought me to,
 the one that started it all.
Red that seeped into my right eye
by a moment of inattention in the schoolyard,
all thanks to the serrated plastic edge of a dragonfly.
That clinic referred us to British Columbia Children's Hospital. It's unnerving to think that without this injury,
I might not have been brought to a clinic or hospital anytime soon, and would have wandered the world of childhood, platelet-less, extremely vulnerable to any physical injury, with no one the wiser, and no diagnosis. I'm grateful that my vulnerability made itself known through this eye injury, rather than blunt force impact to something more vital. The usual "bumps and bruises" of childhood.
In the subsequent months my eye bled into itself repeatedly, so I eventually lost all "useful" vision.
"Total hyphema" refers to complete filling of the eye's front chamber with blood.

In my case, this led to glaucoma and loss of sight.
I don't know when exactly it was that my right eye stopped Seeing.
I don't remember what it's like to see out of both eyes.
I don't miss it. I may as well have been born like this,
were it not for notable intra-ocular pressure.

Intraocular pressure (IOP) is the measure of pressure that has built up within a given eyeball.
Eye pressure is measured in millimeters of mercury (mm Hg).
Normal eye pressure ranges from 12-22 mm Hg,
and eye pressure of greater than 22 mm Hg is considered higher than normal.

After surgery, my doctor notes, my glaucoma-affected eye
was found to be at "a satisfactory 22 mm Hg."
Excellent, I adore being satisfactory.

What the doctors don't mention amongst themselves
is the impact of this intra-ocular pressure on basic quality of life.
IOP causes pain, and when my right eye was in pain,
the signals interfered with the left, the "useful" eye.
I couldn't focus my sight on anything, concentrate,
or, god forbid, hold sustained eye contact.
I felt isolated and alone.

ITP meant I was barred from most forms of physical activity.
IOP meant sleepless nights that bled into fuzzy days and years of ocular shut-in.
At school, sitting in a corner, book in hand, my glaucoma turned me into a Curiosity.

My right eye developed a cloudy white-blue-green colour that I have grown to love in my adult life. Not so, as a child. From the age of 5, when I "lost" my vision, until the age of 16 or so, when I had my last eye surgery, my unseeing eye would regularly keep me up at night in agony until I passed out from exhaustion.

When I was little, Maman and I had a routine:
First, I would scream or whimper, sometime in the evening,
usually around bedtime, when I was already tired
and no longer had the capacity to ignore the discomfort.
Being tired always makes the eye act up, even to this day.
So, I would make known that I was in pain, one way or another,
and try to smother it in a pillow or a series of cold-compresses.
IOP pain feels like my eye is going to explode.
It felt like an ever-inflating ball inside my skull.
I couldn't see out of the offending eye,
so where sight used to be there was only colourful pain.

I kind of understood what was going on,
but that was of little comfort in day-to-day life.
Children have no qualms about
pointing, staring, asking intrusive questions,
venturing patchwork guesses about the nature of someone's difference.
I heard everything from
"your eye grants you oracular powers" (which I like)
to "your eye is that way because someone's cum got stuck in it"
(which fuelled mountains of internalized homophobia)

Kids say stupid things, nothing new here.
Still, it's important for me to acknowledge
how physical difference, especially visible difference from others,
can be deeply distressing as a child.
My visual impairment is a minor disability
that has not gotten in the way of most things I attempt to do in life.
Self-effacing caveat aside,
having a single blind eye
made me a target
of harassment
and bullying
for years.

Sometimes it took the form of a kid hiding around a corner,
waiting to jump-scare me on my blind side
and then lording my inability to see over my head at any opportunity.
Sometimes there were snide comments.
Oftentimes there was no harm meant,
but I still felt myself ever more distant from my peers
as a result of Seeing different and looking different.

Anyone with eyes is likely to agree:
an eye is a very sensitive, delicate ball of goop.
Just as much as eyes are
much-vaunted windows to the soul,
eyes are a means to an end.

In the contemporary north american city, image-saturated,
sight is how I apprehend the world,
it is what I was taught to focus on as the sense of Primary Importance.
Seeing is primordial to Normal Existence,
and eye-contact is how we first build empathy and human connection.
I never regained that much lauded Useful Vision.

By medical standards, my sight is subpar,
and my remaining eye must be protected
(I tend to agree).

Instead of useful vision my stunted optic nerve
reacts to light and dark
picks up on movement
extends my spatial awareness
in ways that differ from seeing.

My right eye won't leave my "useful" left vision alone.
It gets in the way. In my living memory I have never seen double,
but my optic nerve has always kept providing me
with some kind of information.
My right eye does not see, but it feels.
It feels the wind on a cold winter day.
It feels the warmth of direct sunlight like exposed skin.
My occluded, not-useful ball of sense receptors
has maintained hyper-sensitivity to light.
The right eye feeds me never ending waves
of colour and light patterns,
a world of my own

Dreamt

CRYSTAL CLEAR DECIDUOUS DREAMS
where a body uprooted taps
back into the rhizome
Up on the fronds new wings
take flight by attempting
first to fall but find wind
Caught in the bark a beetle
nestles mandibles ever deeper
tunnels and lays the grub

Hum along the chestnut cache
buried where roots gape,
dirt piles with the years.
It's memory that's held in the decay
leaves nothing behind and unturned
sleep remembers a simple moment
Movement, the woodpecker's red crest
staggers to its rhythm. It finds
the beetle hidden, almost.

A swallowed breath hangs
where the beaver decided not to cut:
custodial intelligence is gently exercised.

Excitement builds to a fever pitch
Where the fox spreads its tidings
A party, soon to occur.

Hilarity is a generalized state.
It's happenstance and coincidence
that illusion of unexpected crossings.
Expect less. Open to more.
Scream when it feels right
Not because there's a reason
but maybe there's that, too.

A joy in noise
   Half-friend crossed in the staircase in-out, up-down
   Goes by the name Harriet, kissed
   once at 3am a night of such
   intensity--what was that band
   they always put on? Silver-something?
"Oh, you're not staying for the party?"

Collective understanding develops when I
take it upon myself to voice disagreement.
Similarly: healing is an accumulation of balance
harmony, weight anchored poured molten down
one leg and the other.

Hydration hatchet job
piss yellows then browns
is it the beets
or is it that work gets in the way?
The eyes get too much
when I forget to blink
the neon flickers flash
bulb and to us the nerves
wrecked by artifice, laughable
to be back here after a w/e
of wonder, what the fuck
is this all there is, here.

Of course inward the truth
remains potent, cogent portents
carried upon the wing of a storm
ice falls from the sheet metal roof
wind howls and so I wake up alone
again, my
oh my lover's left for the city.

Apprehend total war
in the neatly packaged dehydrated cheese bites
for sale at the health food store
Where people learn to replace massmarket chips
with ones that come in different plastic.
Instead of waves they crackle
the bag reseals
the asterisk means organic
and I suppose that's a start.

Infinitesimal regression
Industrialism won't loosen its grip
until it's consumed itself to death.
Nothing makes me laugh
when I glimpse through
How am I (lucky enough)
to feel safe in the silence?

She imagines her father
fears nuclear war, maybe
and that's why he stocks
food for winter. As if
there's only one way for supply
chains to collapse.

What speaks vibration tuned
up down the spine its joy
tears well but don't flow here
the freezers wheeze too loud
entirely probable mistakes mean
money comes in when you
Move beyond the absurd need to Do

Wait for it--keep waiting.

What if nothing is still the answer?
Assailed by doubts, here's a reminder:
sitting quietly your friend needs help
gentleness shared, comfort attained for a time.
What is ease, how can effortlessness be?

Nothing nowhere nohow
Merely floating, the rock breaking
the pond's surface tension
sinking the primeval dark
embrace where shadow is honest
Night song the holy dark
Sacrament invented, made up
of those intuitions and traditions
pieced together where
the burrowhole makes itself seen.

Options? Far fewer than you might
expect. Some are true but few
and far between come from
the honest calling. Heartache
melds pain and joy. Know this:
Pragmatics are worth getting settled.

So she laughed at the stars again
like Unju taught her once.
"That's Fomalhaut", they'd say, pointing.
"Remember that name and you'll never
ever be alone." After all this,
the star remains, never condescending,
considered.

And she expected nothing, or less.
Learned at 22 that planning too far
ahead, further than the next season
or so, ultimately leads to ruin. Harriet's
hand struggles with the clay the
pottery wheel in an attempt to subdue
the shape rather than collaborate with
its desire to take form. I'm just
as impatient as I was
back then there, huh? Of course
the difference is recognition. A body
a clay pot, is most potent in its
emptiness.
Does she ever spare a thought
to the depths of the soul?
She claims to sleep at night
unperturbed (by the subtle self)

Consider the locust
swarming, vulpine, initiatic.
I wonder whether she wonders
how many doors she hasn't opened
questioned, knocked up some other
tree, leaves you wondering
how old will she be
when she wakes up to her soul?

Sunlight on the breath. Calm, a high-pitched
silence re-emerges as the mechanical
whirr overheats and halts. First, relief
then a sigh as the diaphragm heaves
up in response to engine failure.
No time to sit quietly at the
now useless controls. There are 12
more acres to be tilled by lunch.
Dry throat, and the nearest tap's
back at home, the bottle on hand's
long empty. So a quenched thirst
needs a fixed engine, and the
engine asks a caring hand not
afraid to rack up the scars
left by hot iron. All this, for
an ear of corn or two.
Father's father told stories of
when corn was maize.

Distill the anxious mind
time is an alembic
through which the fumes focus.
Napping through the winter
solstice to honour the dark
descent's renewal moving into
light the axis shifts
back.

general hilarity as cacao hits the blood
stream of joy, sugar
high, teeter the edge of
inflamed gut brain barrier
and so flatulence ensues
worth every bite, but
glad to be recalibrating
soon enough, later, tomorrow

Theobromine's addictive enough
on its own, and more
with the fats, sugars
from cane, especially.

Your friend is the shared super
organism we all are. Joke's on
the skeptics attending the party
unaware of the fête
all within them

The child knows it is a stone
bouldering at play, playing at
remembering dust of star to
rock, compact, crawling
with moss over quick centuries.

I Reviewed This Nice Boy Whose History You Know Well

ALL THE LETTERS DOCTORS exchanged on the state of my condition in the first few months following my diagnosis have a few things in common. The doctors adopt a formal and clinical tone, getting right to the facts of injury, illness, and treatment. My doctor knows his intended audience:
Other Doctors.
MD to MD.

Why, then, does each letter stress that I was such a nice boy? How is it medically relevant to the treatment of my eyes and blood whether a boy or I'm nice? Getting gendered by medical authority carries weight. Medical sex, as well as gender presentation, seriously impacts how a patient is treated by their doctors.

I have to wonder whether, on the flip side of the gender binary, Dr. C would have referred to me as a nice girl, or added some kind of diminutive? Nice Little Girl, for good measure? I can only speculate, but it seems likely enough. The words we use have everything to do with our environment, and middle-aged men risk carrying subtle hints of misogyny everywhere they go, including their medical practice.

In the treatment of ITP, I can understand how the possession of a uterus impacts treatment after menstruation. What I'm struggling to wrap my head around is why my eye-care specialist felt the need to specify, in each of his letters, that I was a Nice Boy. There's an easy enough explanation: in general, all children get gender assigned, in all walks of life, in a million contexts where it shouldn't matter. This is just one more example of that. Nothing new here. But I'm not satisfied by that answer.

Maybe the language is less stilted than the more clinical The Patient, but it is ultimately less accurate to call me a boy than to call me a patient.

In operation reports, I am The Patient. The function of the documents is the same, isn't it? The letters and the reports? Both provide information about the status of me, Patient/Nice Boy, in order for other doctors to know how things were going with my condition.

The major difference I can pin down stems from whether or not I was conscious during the time period referenced in the document. If I was awake, during a checkup, I was Matthieu-Xavier the Nice Boy. If I was under anaesthetic, during surgery, I became The Patient.

During routine checkups, I had a voice. I answered questions. Shared how I felt, whether I was in any pain. During surgery, I had no feeling, lost all subjectivity. I was asleep. The purpose of our interactions was fundamentally different. From Nice Boy to Patient all thanks to some anaesthetic.

At least Patient stands the test of time. I was only a boy because I'd been told my whole life that I was a boy and didn't know I had the option to disagree, to dissent. I was a boy because terms of endearment like "my little man" have been levelled at me forever. I was a boy because I got Jurassic Park toys and Hot Wheels and Beyblades and those are Boy Toys. I was a boy because I had scruffy short hair. I was a nice boy because I listened to the doctor.

Is the use of Nice Boy a way to show empathy? To acknowledge that I am not only a collection of symptoms, despite what the present letter would otherwise have us believe? By acknowledging my niceness, my boyness, the doctor may be saying:

"This child has a life of some kind
outside our scope of knowledge,
outside of medicine."

To deem me merely The Patient would have reduced my childhood to illness, pathology and nothing else.

To be a Nice Boy in my doctor's letters means he was concerned with my wellbeing.

I remember the ophthalmology wing at BC Children's Hospital in 2001. Those appointments were separate from the ITP checkups. We walked back and forth from oncology. I was at the hospital almost daily that first year.

My eye specialist, Dr. C., who wrote this letter, was a competent doctor and a kind man. Week after week I sat in his examination chair while he prodded my eyes with ophthalmic instruments and did what he could to save my sight. He failed of course, but that was no fault of his. The care proffered by the coalition of doctors and pharmaceutical conglomerates is a tendril of empire.

The doctors convene conferences on autoimmunity.
I imagine they share stories of our bodies'
dysfunctions over cocktails
and look out at the Adriatic sea
from the hotel bar in Athens.

Does the haematologist foot the bill himself,
or does the institution?
Are patients in attendance?

Physicians are on such a pedestal,
all the better to market their expertise in private practice
with such snappy blog-posts as
"14 ways to cure auto-immune disease"
The short of it? Consult with them for 350$/hour.

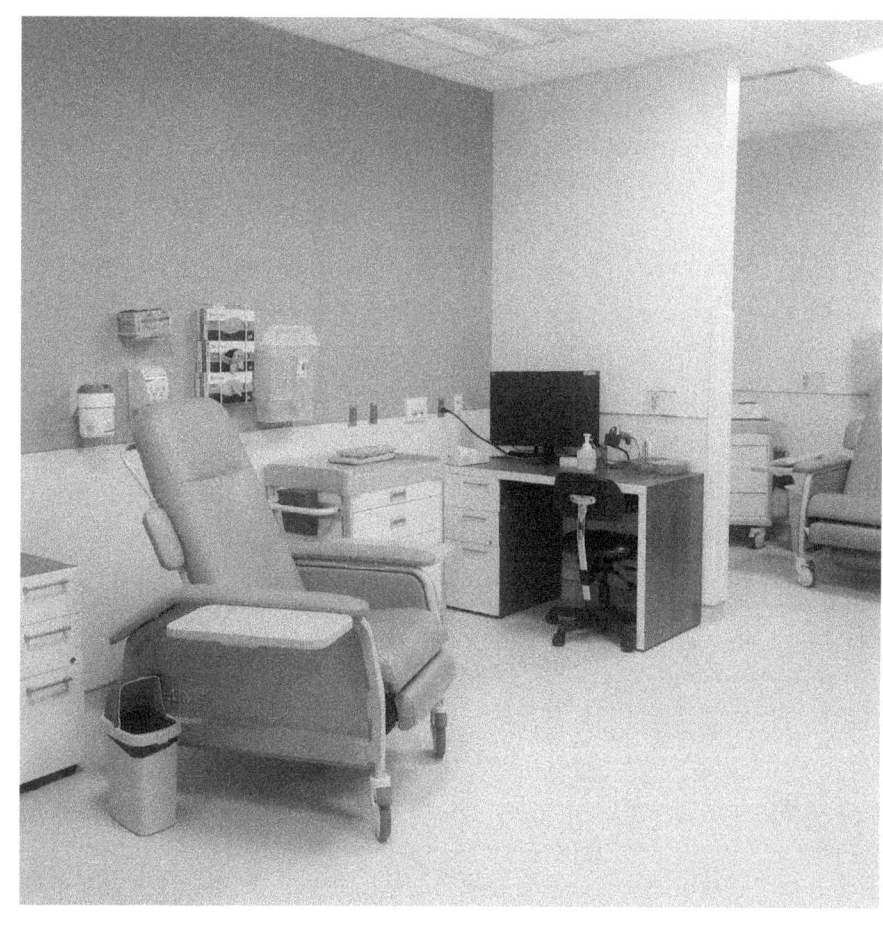

Receiving A Dose

I've got a notion of time crawling
but the room stays the same.
I patiently examine clocks distractions and infusion pumps
as they move and mark different passings.

I use the clock to remind myself clinical purgatory
is impermanent and localized.
While the body sits imbibing the fluid hung from stainless steel
served in pristine glass bottles and gently deflating plastic sacks.

The pump serves to regulate my donor-plasma-derived blood feast,
making sure I don't consume too much, too fast, too little, too slow.
The translucent saline drip opacifies the superstructures
   inherent to (con)temporary cure.

Observing the drip, I easily forget that though the needles seem free,
this watery lifeblood implicates me in the systems I hate.
A cannula is feeding me intravenous immunoglobulin and saline solution.
It was not the first time, it was not the last time.

I am an expert at sitting in hospital chairs
but still have no feeling of power, for my many years of experience.

I've accepted that my doctor knows what my body needs,
   if little else of the world.
World which, outside these clinical walls,
   is rich with joy and sorrow.
But none of that matters now.

Now, I am sitting in a blue chair among blue walls,
bleeding red in purple veins while crystal clear
   plasma fractionations
   make up the difference.

Go on sitting, isn't it comfortable?
Have you ever tried a LUMEX? Best designed chairs around.
Sit for hours in total comfort.
Standard issue LUMEX Clinical Care Recliner,
   designed for blood-work versatility.
Drawing, letting, and transfusing are all viable activities.

As a child I was called a vampire, I embraced it.
I figure a vampire is simply
one who requires liquid supplementation to survive;
one whose blood does not support them on its own;
one whose body is deeply vulnerable
   to specific circumstances.

Receiving intravenous treatment implicates
me in vampiric economic processes
facilitated by biotechnology.
Blood feasts are involuntary, necessary.

Unlike the mythical vampires,
haunting minds and prowling hunting grounds,
my offerings come to me, served up
   through hollow needles handled by steady hands.

Soon afterwards, my body is mine again.
My vampirism is short-lived, if recurrent.
It leaves traces: needle marks, legal restrictions.
My lovers cannot donate blood; I am considered risky.

Combining so many bodies in a transfusion leaves me
brimming with Otherness of the sort blood banks write off.
According to those keepers of frozen life, my blood is impure,
it is a poisonous potion that risks infecting others.

So much of what I consume is involuntary.
Nauseous exhaust, pesticides, heavy metals, microplastics.
I am needfully careful about what I do choose.
A process of elimination, spiraling around a primary principle:
choose what comes from the nearest geographical place,
and which has undergone the fewest transformations.

No coffee, no tea, no chocolate, no refined sugar.
Alcohol depends on the season, and only ever as a food, not an intoxicant.
Cannabis depends on the season,
and is best consumed mixed with other smoking herbs.
Some sources of pleasure, introspection, and social joy.

Vitamins and supplements seem necessary
only because the food that is available for purchase is deficient
in nearly all nutrients. There is a vicious cycle at work,
educating bodies to consume synthetics
rather than what comes from nature.

Prescribed pharmaceuticals are useful, undeniably.
Useful in mitigating symptoms in times of crisis.
But what happens upon habituation?

A chronic treatment engenders chronic illness.
If a body is always consuming synthetic chemicals,
it never learns to heal itself.

Time does not stop, sat in the blue chair, but it does change.
The clock changes, bends to the body's will.
It is the body that determines how long it will take
to fully absorb the dose, how long I will be seated.
Drain the sterile bag of its precious contents
and claim them as part of myself.
It feels like I have no say, I am the witness.
I observe the process and feel the newness within me.
Whose body is it, anyway?

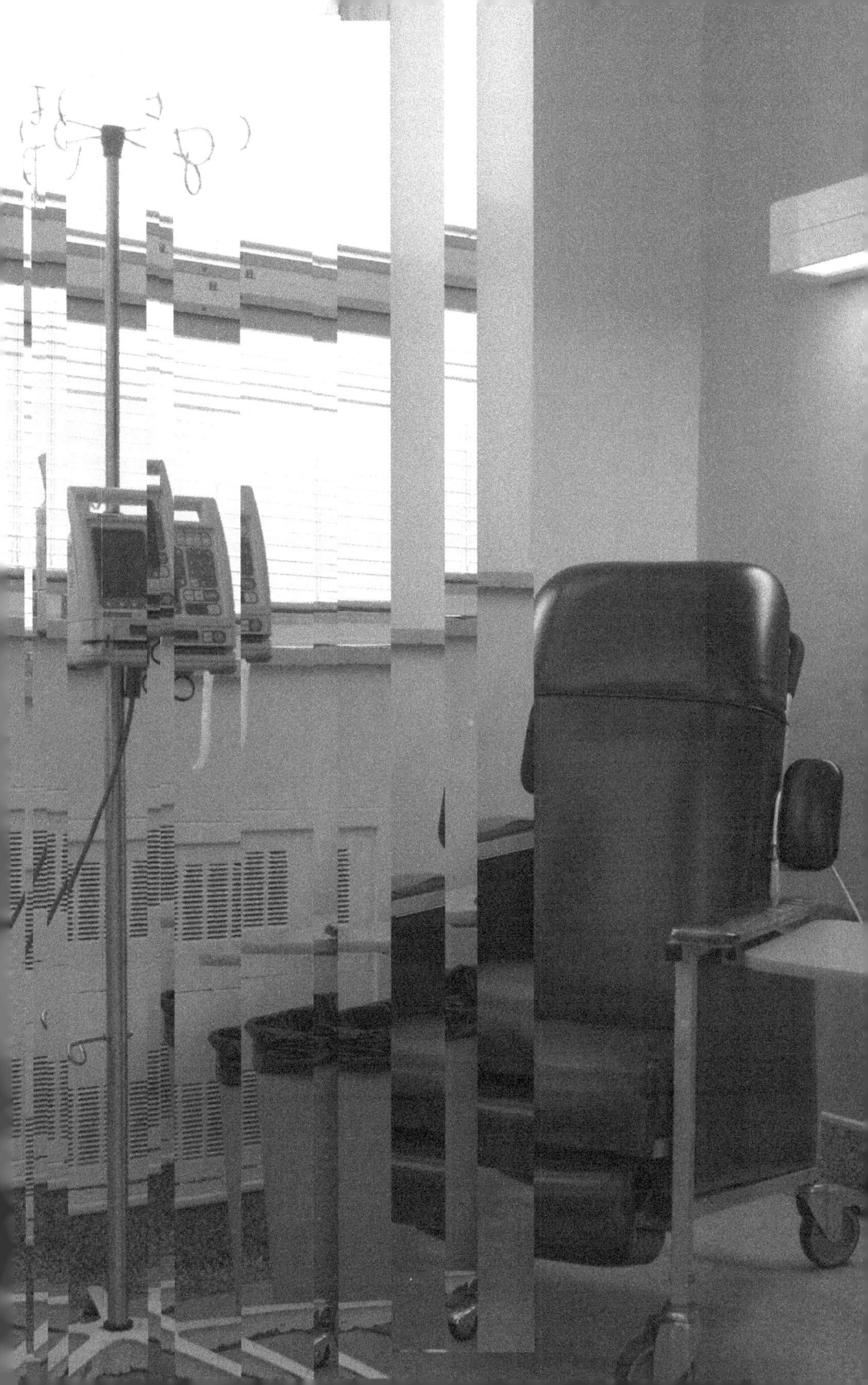

B-12 Adventures

All my body's resources have been somehow drained.
We play catch-up every day of the week, friends.
The able-bodied can hardly conceive this sort of fatigue.
This is not just feeling tired.
This fatigue doesn't care how many hours of sleep I got last night
what I've eaten today, or for my intake of stimulants
This fatigue is the result of a hobbled immune system
swinging its swords at the wrong targets.

Backed into a corner by viral infection, it lashes out.
Not quite at random, but with poor enough aim
that most of my platelets bite the dust at the same time.
My immune system feels like a dormant weapon of mass destruction.

Days get long when your blood is unbalanced.
I've been sitting in a chair all day and still managed a head-rush.
I need to pack more snacks. Seems my anemia is bad these days.
My B12 must be at an all-time low,
considering I've been prescribed a monthly shot.

I've elected to give them to myself this time around.
I do not have enough free time to go to the clinic for a shot every month
when I have the option of doing it at home.
I learned what to do through watching nurses, plus a youtube video.
I've now administered myself the shot 3 times.
The first attempt was a misfire. I froze. I was scared.
Never before had I held a thin metal-tipped
plastic syringe in my own hands.

But I remember being a child playing in the bath
We kept some of the medical syringes used to dose oral drugs
They held a few milliliters of liquid
I used them as water guns in my games.

Now worries swim through my mind:
What if I accidentally contaminated one of the elements of this procedure?
Will I inject myself with bacteria?
What if I inject myself with air?
They say fresh air cures all
but I'm not sure that applies when taken intramuscularly.

So many needles in my life, always in other hands.
So, on the first attempt I scrapped the supplies.
I made it all the way to the part where the syringe was primed with fluid,
needle in my arm, ready to deliver its payload.
I took a few deep breaths, to no avail.
I could not overcome my nerves on that first attempt.

The second time around was a success.
I realized that with my scheduled flu shot coming up,
it was imperative that the B12 be taken before the influenza,
otherwise I would not recuperate from the shot.

This was back in November, during college finals.
So on my way home from my job,
I stopped at the pharmacy and purchased a new syringe
Put 40 cents on my credit card

I got home, and dropped the many
early-winter layers of protection I was wearing
haphazardly around my tiny apartment
in my rush to get the shot over with.

First, I washed my hands, then I gathered up my supplies.
1ml SANDOZ Vitamine B12 1000MCG/ML (DIN 00521515)
which had cost me 8,37$
and had not gone through on the RAMQ public insurance.
Next, generic isopropyl alcohol sterilization pads,
the 1ml syringe, and a finger-shaped Band-Aid™ for afterwards.

I chose the only part of me that has enough fatty tissue,
in order to avoid injecting too deep, and prepared the injection site.
As I approached the needle, it brushed up against one of my fingers.
That was almost enough for me to call it off then and there.
Self-administered shots are nerve-wracking business.
What if I had compromised the needle's sterility
and ended up with blood poisoning?

I took a deep breath, and carried on.
Ultimately unfounded worries.
Before I knew it the needle had been inserted
and the syringe plunger was waiting for its action.

More deep breathing.
In: ready yourself.

Out: slowly contract your left hand's thumb so as to inject the B12 fluid.
Watch it happen in the mirror, hardly feeling,
caught up in breathing, pushing away the fear.
In certain contexts the Bene Gesserit mantra rings true:
Fear is the mind killer.
I feared that I was unable to safely take the necessary steps.
I wanted to defer to a Professional. It boils down to this:
I feared that I hadn't the ability to take care of myself.

That's always the fear when faced with a new challenge.
Will I be able to do what is required in order to continue living?
So far the answer has always been yes.

A Visit To The Blood Doctor

I saw my haematologist (blood specialist) recently.
Well, first, I saw a Resident doctor under his tutelage.
This Resident had an air of confidence in her knowledge,
 seemed nervous holding down the clinic.

As I reported on my recent health and confirmed the information on file, she took simple notes in neat handwriting. She then asked me to wait while she went to speak with my doctor. The young Resident returned with Dr. O, a kindly middle-aged man with whom I have a good working relationship.

He commented that I look well, to go along with my numbers, which have been positive as of late following a tumultuous year. We have the data to back this up: 18 recent blood tests. Not an an all-time yearly high for me, but a respectable amount. Dr. O noted that my hair seemed especially curly.

"You're always reinventing yourself." he quipped.

"Well, I'm young." I replied.

We exchange some pleasant banter. I'm probably one of his younger patients. He's been following my case since I was 19, and has seen me go through a number of phases and changes.

When I first met Dr. O in 2015 I was hospitalized. I had recently moved to Montreal and didn't have a specialist yet. It was my second semester of university, I had overworked myself and caught influenza. He got me sorted out.

That year, I was transfused a few rounds of Intravenous Immunoglobulin (IVIG), which got my platelets to shoot up briefly before plummeting again. There's a lot to be said about this drug, but that's for later. For now, suffice to mention that it's a common treatment for ITP and other medical conditions.

Later that same year, Dr. O got me on a more recent medication, which I still take now (as of writing, in early 2020). Presently, I am prescribed 75mg of Revolade®, manufactured by Novartis Pharmaceuticals Canada Inc. This medication's active component is "eltrombopag", which is a "thrombopoietin receptor agonist."

I have been taking this medication at varied dosages since mid-2015. Its purpose is to act as a productivity coach for my bone marrow, urging it to produce more blood platelets. The pills come in 25, 50, or 75mg compositions of different colours.

I speculate that the pills are different colours because it makes them easily identifiable on the factory floor, so that a 50mg pill has a rather slim chance of finding itself in a packet of 25mg pills.

In fact, I have never seen such a mixup, so I suppose their system is working. No, mixups in dosage have always come from human error on my end. I'm pretty good about remembering to take my meds now. It's baked into my daily routine, but sometimes I'll forget.

Skeletal formula of eltrombopag olamine

I'll be out of the house with plans to
stay elsewhere overnight, and didn't bring my pills.
Or I waited too long before calling the pharmacy
to renew, so I've got none left,
and it's Saturday right now,
and the pharmacy doesn't get any deliveries on Sunday,
so they won't have my Revolade until Monday
because it's a special order.
In 5 years, they've never just happened to already have it in stock.
Again, I'm not certain why that is, but can venture a guess
that I'm one of very few, if not the only person
around here who's got it prescribed.
There's also the matter of cost,
without the RAMQ
or private insurance
footing the bill.
About 4500$ per 28 days' supply.

Thankfully, a yearly bureaucratic process grants me access with minimal monetary expense. If Revolade were not currently my only viable option, I would not be on this drug. Its side-effects & precautions sheet, included in every box, is the size of a poster, with one side in english and the other in french. Some potential side-effects include: cataracts. I can't wrap my head around that one. The prospect of developing cataracts, the implication of going "totally blind", at the age of 20-something, is not appealing. In practice, that's not remotely likely to happen, so I keep taking the drug.

But it's a stroke of luck that I'm fluently bilingual
so that I can get anxious in two languages.

Becoming Sick, Becoming Trans

When I showed a friend some of these writings early on, they said:

> Picturing you as a protagonist on some wild life ride helps me digest the fact that everything you're experiencing is real and at times scary. I think I would worry far too much otherwise. I hope your newsletter allows you to experience some form of escapism, if only for a few fleeting moments. How could you not, with all that imagery?

I replied:
Dear Friend, this is not for me a form of escapism.
- Lately, I've been experiencing feelings that I don't yet have the right language to describe. Some of what I feel is vigour, passion, lust, sorrow, loss. My body feels sore but good, which is an unusual combination for me. I feel connected to the world yet distant. Perhaps most importantly, I feel angry that the world is so many of the ways that it is right now. I feel possessed by rage, which, I'm beginning to realize is at the root of how I choose to be in the world.
- I feel as though the quote-unquote "sickness" that has shaped my life is little more than a cultural fiction. I do not mean narrative fiction with political themes. Someone reading a novel or a story can close the book and leave the realm of fiction behind. There is an important difference between cultural fiction and narrative fiction.

Cultural fiction is the realm of lived experience formed by all our received notions of what is and is not possible in reality. It feels as though the words I've used to describe myself over the course of my life are becoming increasingly senseless. Cultural fiction is the language I learned to use to identify myself with people, groups, categories. Name, sex, gender, political status.

"How about we all go around and introduce ourselves?

Let's do names, pronouns,

and anything else you feel like sharing."

All of these words are useful short-hand for use on official documents. For many people whose legal identity markers differ in ways from mine, these words are necessary for survival, for recognition and access to essential community and services. These Words are not identity. I believe there is no essential identity, only a shifting set of relations, many of which determine social-political status. I use words regularly in order to access medication, credit, lodging; they remain political fictions. The same system which designates me as Male leads to my diagnosis as Chronically Ill, a nice boy. Politically, I am my "deficient" immune system as much as I am a male of legal voting age. In actuality, I am not Matthieu-Xavier Marin, though that is the name that appears on my passport. I echo here Paul B. Preciado's words:

I am not a man and I am not a woman and I am not heterosexual I am not homosexual I am not bisexual. I am a dissident of the sex-gender system. I am the multiplicity of the cosmos trapped in a binary political and epistemological system.

For me, being trans is being sick and being sick is being trans. I do not seek medical/legal transition. My gender (or lack thereof) and my political identity are as real as my illness. My body is already the product of modern medicine, official Womanhood does not call out to me. My body has been the blood of unknown thousands worldwide, it was the Penicillin I took for over a decade, and is the anti-haemorrhage pills I take every day now. I do not want or need synthetic estrogen to cease being Male, I have long since been in transition. My body has been in revolt against the sex-gender system from the moment my immune system went haywire and began attacking its host: Me.

The moment a twist of fate blinded one of my eyes I was no longer the Male fiction which was assigned to me at birth, I was (and am) A Patient. And now, I am learning how to cope with the dis-identification from masculinity, sickness, and health. There is no escaping these fictions which shape my body and yours. Every time I go to a clinic I reaffirm the fiction that is Matthieu-Xavier Marin, the fiction of masculinity, the fiction of Immune Thrombocytopenia, all in order to receive treatment which increases my quality of life.

When the power to withhold treatment may be so quickly brandished, I act counter to my beliefs. If medicine could treat bodies without gendering them, if it were possible to be considered a sovereign political subject without necessarily being M or F, millions of people would not share my problem. In the current binary system, it is not possible. Honestly, not undergoing Official Transition is a form of harm reduction, of not making more friction for myself.

In naming these things as fiction, I do not deny their material reality. But new fictions must be invented in order to account for the multiplicity of experience.

I write it in order to speak. I am writing to engage in dialogue. I am writing with others to redefine what is possible, in order to bring new versions of myself into existence. This is an enactment of who I am in the world. It is my way of playing with language until I can find out how to describe and share what my reality consists of. I am speaking the death of my sick human body, and of the fictions which have shaped my worlds, in all the complexity that entails. All this, in order to better imagine new possibilities for existing with each other.

Photophobia and Blind Gain

Transcription of doctor's letter, 2001:

Dear Dr. B, RE:M-X MARIN.

Further to my previous letter regarding this nice little boy, we have continued to follow him up on a weekly basis. Matthew has becomes very light shy. His examination is quite difficult as a result. Slit lamp examination on the right shows profound corneal staining which has worsened since he had a further bleed inside the right eye. On the left sight, the slit lamp examination is difficult.

Nevertheless, I was able to obtain a good view of his cornea, anterior chamber, iris, lens and anterior vitreous. There is no suggestion of ocular inflammation whatsoever. His corneal surface is intact and there is no conjunctival inflammation either. I cannot account for Matthew's symptoms of photophobia. I do not think this is evidence of sympathetic ophthalmia. There is a potential risk of this in view of his past history. I have suggested that he continue to use the topical Voltaren and Prednisolone 1% drops previously prescribed to the right eye and that he re-attend in three weeks. I would like to see him sooner if his symptomatology worsens.

Kindest regards.

According to Wikipedia community editors, Photophobia is an abnormal intolerance to visual perception of light. It is an experience of discomfort or pain to the eyes due to light exposure or physical sensitivity. When my eye doctor diagnosed my photophobia, they were basing themselves on how I reacted to the bright directional lights used for examination.

The word photophobia can also mean morbid fear of cameras or seeing.

It is aversion, an impulse to recoil from looking.

In my regular life, photophobic days are when I won't make eye contact, leaving the house is less likely to happen, and I can't concentrate on anything.

Photophobia is not unlike a migraine. It's kinda like seeing multicolour TV static on those old bunny-ear sets. Over the years, I had a few eye surgeries to diminish eye-ball pressure. Back when the pressure was extremely high, I'd have photophobic days a lot. Lately it's uncommon.

The only cause I've been able to pinpoint for photophobia in my adult life is fatigue. When I am tired, my eyes hurt. A straightforward formula. Following months working full-time at a computer, my tolerance to screens has diminished significantly, so I rarely watch TV anymore.

When my eyes are in pain, I use them differently. I'm not equipped for navigating life without sight, I lack practice. Still, my eyes ask that I take a break from staring into the world, and learn other ways of understanding.

How about another reading of photophobia: not as pathological aversion to sight, but as revolt against vision by Blindness, as "blind gain." I am inspired by the d/Deaf studies narration of deaf gain rather than hearing loss. Deafness and Blindness have been thought of as framing experience. Okay. Whose frame? Who's doing this framing?

Framing is a partial, banal, and unimaginative metaphor about sight. It restricts possibilities outside of "useful vision" by constructing borders around possibilities for constellation. "Looking" appears as just a tool for knowledge. Unfortunately, this tool is weaponized.

Sight is a basis of pathology: it creates normality, symptoms.

Sight bores into reality, to prove it can be seen.

Vision is a scope for framing reality in your sights, making reality a visible entity open to calculation and marketing. I'm so tired of being marketed at. Vision is predatory, capturing images for language to narrow down by force. Looking has been used to choose the visible and construct the invisible. It is mobilized to create fear.

Before one surgery a nurse applied anesthetic goop
to your left hand where the IV would go later.
I didn't protest but soon after the solution began acting upon the nerves
I realized your hand was on its way to disappearing.
I had learned not to trust your eyes
even as they assured us the hand remained visible.

Looking is a trap. Looking occurs from the outside in.
Peering upon the surface of skin of paper of the fire
we see only the surface the folds of visible material.
Gazing at you is accompanied by the inner sense
of flow of blood of breath the pulse if our attention is tuned.

What is the obsession with microscopy?
Tired extension of the eye's desire to sense
surfaces across new territories.
Holders of a pair of human eyes cannot
then be content with the sight
proffered by you my darling the mostly sighted?

For years we glued your eye to a viewfinder
in the hopes of discovering a new way to capture light.
Too late, far too late. The image catalog is overflowing as it is.
Okay, we said, and turned the camera on ourself,
on you, to reshape and mold in static frames what motion only confused.
Day and night rearranging that bedroom above Boul. St-Jo
to catch the sunlight the lamplight against the blank walls,
dreaming of a "real" studio, hardly realizing that
space is not what makes the photograph but indeed it is the eye.
Friends asked how I do it and I quipped
that your singular sight holds many secrets.
That's still true, but photography with its focus on the visible
cannot capture the ocular sublime of your optic nerves.

Photos serve to explore you
to find other angles the mirror doesn't allow,
to rip out your eye and relocate it
6 feet away where the machine holds the key
to new territories of fleshy surfaces
enfolded as we find more positions to reveal you
and put you on display, on a pedestal of our choosing.

Let's understand symptoms of vision loss as blind gain,
in a conscious shift away from the regime of vision.
Blind gain is looking's move beyond instrumental sight.
Blind gain surpasses sight in order to reveal
an invisible present within the ongoing moment.
Blind gain is the feeling that we have much to learn from sightlessness.

It is a sensitivity to the harms enacted by vision.
It is a category for imagining beyond sight.
It is an awareness that a shift in perception is a good thing.
My blindness is always changing.

How come I was told all my life that I had lost vision,
    rather than gained blindness?
Some summer days, my blind eye can take the full brunt of the sun.
Other days, a dim room or my phone's screen
are enough to force both my eyes closed in defence against the light,
so vision can't really look at anything either.
These are those photophobic days, when blindness revolts.
Blind gain creates interference.
The pictures might come through, or not.
Knowledge is open to all, and images are not life.
To feel deeply, we must think beyond the visible.
The sensation of flows in my body is enough proof that I am still alive.

AUTO-IMMUNE HERESY

I am troubled by our senses, and sight's legacy within feeling.
We tend to impose perception rather than feel with honesty.
"Framing" so much as the birds we may hear or the earth we lay on.
Verily, enframing is sight's doing, vision's call to arms.
Framing restricts fields of experience, like we have long penned animals:
to keep them in sight, under relative control.
Frames are borders: geometric and geographic,
    imposed by the Eye's vision.
Framing establishes a relationship of domination
    between parties meeting upon the field.
Given that sight is essentially limited, it seeks unseen territories
in order to deepen, widen, and stratify its expanse.

Sight is a tool, wielded by Power, so that previously-unseen
others may be ensnared and dispossessed by its frames.
Sight is a barometer of what is allowed within or without,
as human or other, white or other,
man or other, straight or other, living or dead.
Sight lacks nuance, even in its waning imperial rule.
Sight is the trouble we stay with even while learning about alternatives.
We're stuck with it, as seers or seen and often as both.

Transgressive is any act which would break down the frames
and create unseen realms of possibility.

Blind gain is an unframing, an unseeing, a re-realizing without borders,
where we may share with each other what we know and
what we might use.

0 1 MARS 2019
0 3 JAN. 2020
0 9 AVR. 2019
2 3 AVR. 2019
2 9 MAI 2019
1 1 JUIN 2019
1 1 JUIL. 2019
2 5 JUIL. 2019
1 5 AOUT 2019
2 9 AOUT 2019
1 2 SEP. 2019
2 7 SEP. 2019
1 1 OCT. 2019
2 5 OCT. 2019
0 8 NOV. 2019
2 2 NOV. 2019
0 6 DEC. 2019
2 0 DEC. 2019

Sickness As A Way Of Life

2020-04-01

SICKNESS INVOLVES LEARNING HOW the body is remedied and poisoned.

When sickness and medicine come together, they create illness. Living well with an ever-present awareness that sickness exists is a learned practice. I learned as I grew up in-and-out of hospitals.

I am reading The Immune System, A Very Short Introduction, because I do not understand how how the body's biology works. I'm finding this Introduction scientifically informative, but I've got a bone to pick with its language.

As an example, the book's metaphor for viral infection is of "hijacking" cells. To me, that language implies that our cells are private property being commandeered by a virus and driven off course towards doom. This rhetoric of the body seems to make our own bodies unworthy of trust. They must be controlled, bridled like wild horses.

Different bodies have different claims to ownership, and enact varying degrees of violent repression

to maintain ownership over the cells of other bodies. For a Citizen in 21st century so-called-canada, which I am, the ownership-bid is divided up in as many parts as there are calls for us to work productively, or encouragements to consume "freely" the fruits of global economic production shipped to our northern land. This is a soft repression.

In Illness as Metaphor, Susan Sontag dissects the literature concerning Tuberculosis and Cancer. Pervasive disease of the 18-20th centuries. She finds that a recurring metaphor for Turberculosis is "consumption." Consumption is defined here as a manner of appearing ill. It was envisioned glamorously. Many aristocrats adorned themselves "consumptively." Tuberculosis was fashionable.

For others in Sontag's analysis, consumption was viewed as a habit to be broken. In other words: the malady of Tuberculosis itself was a habit. In all cases, Sontag's metaphors of illness seem concerned with the perception of illness in others, with its representation after the fact, not with the lived reality of sickness.

Sontag herself had 3 cancers, and died with the third. She never published auto-biographical texts in her life. But I took a detour to read her early journals, 1947-1963. Poor Susan had no grasp on her emotions. She is ruled by them even as she parses out the intellectual intricacies of life. These journals take us from ages 16-30 or so. From auditing classes at Berkeley, through marriage, early years of her child David, bohemia in Paris, and life as a young writer in NYC. She's struggling throughout with How to Love, Be a Jew, Be a Writer. She reads widely and ceaselessly. Voraciously considers her culture, lives it. All the while, the journals are precipitously self-conscious. "How do I exist?" A perpetual reflexive self-analysis. Relentless. Sontag never once relaxed in all these 15 years. Her love affairs all strike me as childish. Why? She is entrapped, stuck in co-dependency. She admits in the 60s that she feels rarely able to be alone, that she feels un-self-sufficient. She vampirized her lovers. No doubt some of that was mutual, but as a reader I saw only S.S' view. As a reader indeed, the experience was thrilling. The sheer intimacy of it. I dreamt of her last night.

Somehow, the ill are read as on their way to death's door. Sontag's book was reviewed as an exhilarating "literary" performance, in spite of her explicit point that "illness" is not a metaphor. She was wrong. Susan would have us regard illness in a "healthy" way "purified" of metaphoric thinking. Simultaneously, she enforces borders between "Kingdoms of health and ill." It seems that, to Sontag, illness broke life into a binary Good and Bad. 40 years later, those alleged borders are radically porous. Each of us harbours a near-constant awareness that at any moment we may fall ill and be rendered dependent on others for our ability to consume. Sickness demands that we trust the people around us.

What does it mean, to trust?
How can we trust our own bodies,
let alone others,
when a virus is pandemic?
How could we possibly trust,
when we understand viral infection as an attack,
a virus as a combatant?
When we're always on the defence, shields raised?
Instead of virus as hijacker, what about the virus as teacher?
From a virus, a host body learns to develop anti-bodies with which to eliminate the infection.

How many of us now are now unsure what to do with our days,
when we can hardly produce or consume?
How many of us feel guilty?
This moment is an opportunity to learn other ways
of using time and resources.
How many of us are afraid?
How can we defend ourselves against the metaphors of illness and viral infection at once?
Illness is an idea, and it is shaped by how we invoke the word.
Illness is the stress, fear, restlessness, guilt, and unease we are feeling.
Illness is why many of us don't know what to make of their days.

Sickness as a way of life is an ecology of presence,
an acceptance of the covenant between our bodies and the earth.
We alive now are not any more guilty for pandemic than climate change,
but we must be responsible for how we respond to both and more.

Populations have been violently dispossessed of responsibility by the dominant order of things,
and we are at grips to reclaim our presence on the living earth we inhabit.
Pandemic may serve as disillusionment within apocalypse.
We are here. Not morally or legally bound to responsibility,
but filled with desire to promote renewal, reciprocity, and respect.
This moment is so full of embodied potentials.

Time flows by. Saturdays, I am not turning on my phone or computer.
How much physical isolation is by design? How are 'safety' and 'productivity' linked?
Pandemic is globally a herald for martial law. Public safety restricts interpersonal contact to forms dictated by law so that 'unsafe' actions may be limited. Organizing mass physical protest seems unthinkable when pandemic is rampant. The imposition of public safety over history has forced acts of public revolt to assume non-violent forms. "Peaceful protest." With increased surveillance came increased reliance on subterfuge. There was a move away from violent uprising toward ideological battle. Peoples were dispossessed of arms so that power may keep them. The disarmament of society and the militarization of policing co-operate with the word of law to ensure "safety."
We rely on ideas to keep us safe rather than the bodies we inhabit, so we have no more arms with which to care for ourselves. How can we take responsibility if no one has taught us how? It is a matter of learning how to be sick.

Sickness is a call to collective action.
Sickness is what families, communities, and affinity groups come together to care for.
Sickness is a way of life.
Illness is sickness' ethic reduced to a pathology.
Illness is a means to shrug off personal responsibility.

It removes us from the lived reality of sickness all around.
My sickness is real enough.
Real, in that doctors have a name for it.
A set of treatments. An agreed-upon scale of severity.
Real in fact because it is named, and quantifiable.
Little guesswork remains, there are the facts, the diagnosis.
Illness, still, is obscene.

In conversation, I notice people seem afraid to utter the word pandemic.
A rock-star academic already has a book about COVID-19 available for pre-order.

I feel like a teenager, back when everything was "so sick",
even while illness had long enveloped the entirety of my waking life.

Every day, I question: what is worth doing right now?
Currently Reading, Writing, Talking, Walking, Dancing,
Cycling, Tai chi, Qi-Gong, Meditating, Cooking, Sleeping,
Playing and Watching by myself and with myself, Photography
are all worth doing for me.

I have learned that an excess of self-discipline is no substitute for spontaneity and joy,
so I smoke cannabis because it helps me feel better and more contemplative.

I live alone with support, and I am screen-averse.
This is a difficult combination right now,
when a breach in loneliness comes mostly through the internet.

I have felt guilty for my own improved well-being amidst pandemic.
How is it that I should feel in may ways
better than two weeks ago?
So many others are suffering right now.
Yet I have more energy, more willpower,
and a renewed sense of purpose.
Daily my desire to create grows.
I feel more present in the world now than I ever have.

The apartment I rent houses me alone.
I do not wake up or sleep near others right now.
My days are mostly devoted to contemplation.
I am supported in making sure my material needs are met.
For me, the radical slow-down of daily life
has been a deeply positive thing.
My awareness of current-global-events has narrowed.
I only really follow certain local developments.
I know the rest of the news-cycle exists too,
but since I don't seek it out,
it rarely comes to me by accident.

Staying around my home and limiting commercial contact
has allowed me to devote far more time to resting.

Doesn't anyone else find Rest difficult to come by when daily routine involves commuting and working among hundreds and thousands of others? The press of city life is exhausting and driven by an excess of accumulation and commerce.

It's honestly far more pleasant to stay home.
Here, I feel control over the ideas that direct my life.
I can unplug my clock, and suddenly time is radically changed for me.
The mot-d'ordre ceases to be.
I'm suddenly aware my rhythm is in tune with the rising and setting sun,
rather than the numbers on the dial.

You Matter
2020-04-08

I LIVE FOR MYSELF. How could it be any other way?

I am selfish. I acknowledge that within my own life, my wellbeing comes first. It is by keeping myself alive that I can best support others. Those I love, who turn to me for support, I want to be there for them. If I do not do what I must in order to feel good and whole within myself, I cannot sustainably support others. Our lives, intertwined, I do not wish them extirpated, no matter what the government regulations stipulate. I want to enmesh us further, to know what comes of closeness. To do this, we must learn when to say 'No. Enough. Not right now.'

This is not up to authority to determine, it is individual responsibility. So long as I am able, I will turn this ability into good. I am no better or worse than anyone else. Each of us is here, and learning what that means. How can anyone possibly presume to know what's best for another person? We all have different answers. I tend my own garden and share the harvest. I strive to glean carefully what each world-fragment has to share. To recognize and shed prejudice, gather each thing on its own as a whole part of the larger universe.

Daily I take stock of my capacity. Variability and fluctuation unlike ever before. Or perhaps I'm just more perceptive. I've been in a more personally tumultuous state before. Now, the tumult is outside. My inner life is relatively calm. I notice its intricacies in more detail, it is with both apprehension and excitement that I write down my dreams. I aim to Stop expecting a text back. Stop demanding a response. Each of us is overwhelmed by demands on our attention. Forget any notion that you are more important than any one else. I am not any more important than anyone else, don't get back to me if you don't have the energy, and please do not feel guilty. Everyone on earth, without exception, is part of what is underway ever after this state of limbo.

Share what matters to you, far and wide, regardless of expectation. Make no demands on the energy of others unbidden, but do not be afraid to share. What is it that is keeping you going right now? No matter how benign, someone else empathizes. Our ideas must flow with compassion. We feel the way together.

How do I feel? I feel my feet cocooned in thin socks, intimately familiar with the old wood floor. I know the floor's dips and inclines, for having stood alone with it. I feel my window facing 120 degrees SE, if my dusty old compass is to be believed. I feel the sun's rays rising through the southeasterly portal. I've cracked it open, so I'm stroked by spring breeze and I hear spring sound. I feel excitement and determination, as I focus on my projects.

I feel the air I breathe, and I feel the tightness of anxiety in my lungs.

I feel both my eyes distinct from one another.

I feel the nerves sprouting from the skull's base, connecting me.

I see the sun on my skin and sense pleasant warmth.

I bear a light ache in my heart as sad thoughts of distant separation come to mind.

I pause, and read a paragraph from Phèdre aloud to myself.

Unable to digest more than that at once, I lay the book back down on my desk.

Plato's Socrates is opposed to allegorical interpretation of the world.

Following the Oracle at Delphi's guidance, he chooses to focus on learning himself.

And who do I presume to be? One whose voice rings clear within the depths of my own flesh. A body is anything but transparent, I contain far more than the sum of my parts. Each action I take for my own wellbeing drives me forward toward a higher version of myself. Completing even the most benign tasks is part of the puzzle. Self-care is primordial. I love this world. I love existing with/in it. I love its simplicity and complexities. The wellspring of sensation runs deeper than I can ever know. All my efforts to feel deeply spiral together, sharper and deeper, plunging my body into itself. I leave aside preconceptions about what it is possible for me to feel, and take new/familiar sensations as they come, not disbelieving my own grasp of reality. Why should I ever tell myself a feeling is false? I am blessed with an honest body, one which attempts no trickery. It is with time and patience that I learn the grammar of sensation. There is no formula for love, there is only acknowledgement of its possibility and dedication to its practice. Love is a choice.

Inner life is inherently true, there is no contradicting solipsistic experience. Inner life risks becoming false when it butts up against the outer world and its many contradictions, yet the truth of inner life does not make it serene. Truth can be chaos, hurt, confusion. It is through acceptance that I begin to make sense of my truth. Facing unpleasant truth is difficult. It's much simpler to focus only on positives, to live as though everything ought to be pleasurable all the time. Even now, there are so many positives.

Focusing on pain is a necessary means of better understanding my place in the world, my relationship to my past, my needs in the present, and my desire for a future. Not those material wants which lend themselves to a certain lifestyle, but the needs of which drive me.

So many questions from disparate sources with ongoing answers: What is the capacity for violence? What do we harness, to grow in power? Who are we? How can we be meaningfully frightened? What happens when the temporarily-able-bodied, the not-ill, begin to roam again? What is the value of escape in living with presence? How do we balance Here+Now with Then+There in order to survive pandemic's emotional toll? What is it about stories of unreal proportions that feel so liberating?

Storytelling is freedom-making. The reading of stories is a cure for loneliness and it is an amnesiac. Reading is a matter of embodying the reality suggested in the text. There is a great beauty in this temporary commandeering of memory. Give up on courage, and escape. How wonderful, that I might ignore human suffering for a time, and empathize with narrative fiction instead. Draped in its own fictions, waking life hurts me to bear. So much is wrong and so much is uncertain. In re-reading a familiar story, I can suspend my knowledge of how much I do not know here and now, to indulge in knowing some future, and strap into the tumult leading up to an ending.

For there is an end, even to 3000 page sagas. The printed page is floriously static. It does not risk slipping into new terrifying realms of as-yet-unimagined unknowns. I have picked a narrative I know, I am familiar with the arc upon which I will fly. And there, escaping into other identities, I find comfort.

There is no going back to normal.

Normal?

Normal as in healthy?

There can be no going back because what pandemic reveals is the fiction of health. We have never been healthy. Health is a story woven by institutional power in order to create a reality in which it is possible to negate certain lives on the basis of abnormality or pathology.

Pandemic extends the logic of medicalization to everyone. Prevention is currently the treatment preached by the government of canada, so that we may slow the spread of COVID-19 and not overwhelm our public healthcare infrastructure. The infrastructure relies on previous expectations of how many might fall ill at a given time, and the built environment reflects that calculus. The status of illness in society is undergoing radical change, as we all now may be sick. What does it mean to be considerate of fellow humans, living in close quarters?

It's 5 in the morning, I'm up, as usual,
and the neighbours below me are singing.
I don't think they slept.
It seems they waited to hear footsteps before breaking out the guitar.
They've belted soft melancholy into the early dawn.
I feel the floor rumble beneath my feet.
It's early, but then, there is no too early for music.
It is a matter of body-clocks, social-clocks, unplugging digital clocks.
My neighbours doubtlessly need this music now,
though most of us are quiet at this, the last hour before sunrise.
I cannot reproach them their joy and their camaraderie as it rubs off on me.
Sing another song, boys.

Digressions
2020-04-17

> Need the success of a political group be measured on its impact on a larger social order?
> — Dodie Bellamy

Why not a change of pace
whats the point of
habit it's just learned
unlearned re:re:re:
me me me who's to
say really it never
was about me it is
about them and us
what would you do
you who one day learned
to hold a pen read their
words right about now
new words new pens
to stab with lances
megaphones canons leaking
ink sapping energy
sporadic like forests spreading
there goes the love of my life
meat smells meld of wills.

Active mecha-thoughts span soma-
thèques disjointed rapiecé rafistolé
Un Deux Trois how many of me
Do I think cohabitate? It's a non-issue
really doesn't matter scatter
my ashes to the wind they got
caught in a web cautiously
woven silken threads so inviting
me to rest amidst delicate
morning dew Who? You heard her
left right and deep time
out take a break down this
imaginary wall it's not so tall
we can jump it if we
strap dynamite to our chairs
and say hold on to me darling
Dream loud if at all
They have the most beautiful
eyes, non? Yes oui magnifique
Hold the staring contest pit up
a photograph guaranteed victory
frozen snapshots longing joyous
Hours of liquid poured down
honeyed throats.

38.5 degrees centigrade
2020-04-22

When I have a fever and my temperature reaches 38.5C, I go to the hospital. Usually, best practice while experiencing fever is to let the body sweat itself out. Fevers are a natural broad-spectrum defence mechanism, very effective, just stay hydrated. For me, best practice is not to let the fever run its course, because a fever contains too many unknowns. Coronavirus has brought fever into sharp relief as a symptom. Fever, for all its utility, is a source of fear.

September 2001

I am the first laparoscopy-splenectomy patient
at BC children's hospital in Vancouver.
For half a chance of inducing ITP remission,
I undergo surgery to remove my spleen.
Laparoscopy is a minute procedure consisting
of many small incisions
for the entry of surgical tools;
cameras, suction tubes, knives.
It's an alternative to open gut surgery
with less obvious marks left on the body's surface.
Your scars are barely noticeable
if you don't know to look,
or if fingers aren't searching.
The procedure separates surgeon from patient with a camera,
extending the careful eye for steady hands.

Doctor doesn't get to peer directly
into patient and examine the organs firsthand,
must trust that the camera feed
is an accurate depiction of the body.
And why wouldn't it be?

The lens and the sensor are trusted
sources of fact, or so the story goes.
Biologically, the spleen is a sort of filter for blood.
It's not all that vital until you get an infection,
at which point it is a very useful line of defence.
Spleen removal is a common treatment
for Immune Thrombocytopenia,
because the spleen occasionally destroys too many platelets.
For me, it induced a partial and temporary remission
that left me taking oral penicillin tablets
daily to kill off infectious bacteria.
(no one thought back then of antibiotics abuse, overprescription)

When I was little I couldn't swallow the pill
so maman crushed it up with a mortar and pestle
I swigged it with orange juice, juice or water,
got a treat afterwards.
Gummy bears. Positive Reinforcement.
Doctor's Orders Better Safe Than Sorry.
Despite the antibiotics, we regularly rushed
to the hospital in the middle of the night.
The problem with not having a spleen
is the speed at which an infection might turn deadly.
That's why, when I have a fever of 38.5C I go to the ER.
Usually it's just the flu.
When my immune system starts doing its job
— eliminating infection —
it also remembers just how much
it despises my blood platelets.
The result is that any infection
leaves me with dangerously low platelet counts,
sometimes in the range of
"may spontaneously bleed internally."
I am not afforded the possibility of waiting it out
and seeing whether my condition improves on its own.
Yeah odds are it's fine i'll just sleep it off
but what if it isn't?

H1N1, 2009

I didn't get the vaccine
and wasn't alive for the 1918 outbreak.
No antibodies, so I catch swine flu late June.
40C fever near delirious in Ottawa children's hospital bed,
I remember my friends were on a school trip to Toronto
strapped in to roller-coasters at an amusement park to experience excessive g-force.
I may have played video games, I'm not sure, I don't remember.
I created my first Runescace account in 2006, I was 10 years old. I'd play in the couple hours waiting for test results before the doctor's visit. I think I found it because it was popular on Miniclip. The soundtrack, the world, the slow pace; Runescape is a waiting game. I remember discovering my player character's limits heading West, followed by an in-game pal. "Where are we going?" "To find the elves." --only, the elves are pay-walled. Eventually, I convinced Maman to pay my membership fee, but I never progressed through to the elven settlement. A simple structure: Quests, levels, trading, combat. Goals to reach. Power to gain. Every attainment felt hard-earned in its reward. The community, active and friendly back then, seemed to be composed mostly of other kids around my age. Now, I guess it's probably mostly adults on a nostalgia trip.
The point-and-click adventure in waiting. Waiting for the trees to grow. Waiting for adversaries to spawn, waiting for mineral ore to appear in the rocks. RS' world is scaled up to a speed that keeps players waiting, but not too long. Not so long that progress feels halted. Cycles are quick enough for us to sit at the computer with baited breath, eagerly awaiting the next clic. And what's more, it a resource is too crowded, a hundred parallel worlds are available.

Waiting can be circumvented. The player is afforded enough control and power that the actions in game feel like meaningful progress.

It is the ideal game for limbo.

In pandemic, 4 friends and I got back into the game. "I've always wanted access to this content" says one about the members-only stuff. Now a work-from-home graphic designer, what better way to escape the condo of the 50th floor above Toronto than into Gelienor? The so-called real-world is stuck, we have no control, so the desire to make progress is well-suited to the game.

Runescape accomplishes nothing useful. And how glorious, that nothing is productive. No personal growth, no professional development, no upskilling. It can be said that playing an MMORPG is refusal to capitalize on leisure time. A queer use of time; failure to behave. Simple indulgence in a designer world with quantifiable barometers of progress that are attainable to any player willing to put in the necessary time.

I probably played it during my H1N1 infection, too.

Summer 2012

a lethal heatwave sweeps north America
but Maman and I are on vacation in Europe.
I think it's the second or third time I'm over there
I'm having fun but I miss my girlfriend.
In Paris I took lots of rainy pictures
with a camera my high school teacher lent me for the summer.
We leave Paris by TGV to Montreux, Suisse.
After a couple of days in bourgeois paradise
we drive up to visit friends in Château-d'Œx,
famous for its Balloon Week.
I'm fine when we set out on the road
but after lunch I start feeling ill
and am feverish by the time we make it
to Maman's friend's home.
We think I'm just tired so I go to sleep
after taking a picture.

Description of Image taken in the Swiss alps, July 2012:

Foreground of verdant field leading up to a large wooden cabin overlooking a hill, with bright green window shutters open but windows closed and white curtains pulled. Further afield on the other side of a second grassy hill, dense forest hugs the mountain slopes partially lit by sun as cloud-shade cuts across. Background of mountainous peaks sparsely wooded against cloudy sky of cotton-candy clouds.

I don't have a solid grasp of how much time passes.
I play that old Pandemic 2 flash game
in a fever haze on a slow ethernet
connection in the swiss alps.

Something catches my eye on screen
Virtual September 2008:
 - first victim dies in china
 - china begins burning bodies to prevent infection.
I take a screenshot,
highlight the back-to-back event dialogs,
make a post ironically titled
"Boy, that escalated quickly"
and get 537 comments.

My bedsheets are changed regularly as I sweat profusely
the adults decide it's time to get me to a hospital
when blood shows up in my stoole.
The friend we're staying with is a healer.
One afternoon I sit shivering across from her and we talk.
She peers into my 15 year old eyes and
reveals to me my own fear of death.
She doesn't have the medicine to stop the bleeding
but we hug and I feel impending doom leave my body
in a rush of cathartic relief
I'm hyperventilating
my lips quiver like my pulse is wholly
contained in that patch of split pink
I can't speak I try to breathe
my head rushes with light and the world implodes.
I come back to my body slow and suddenly I'm aware
of sunshine through wide windows in a room full of books.
Maman and I take a small mountain train back to Montreux
it's a beautiful day and I devote my time
in peaceful delirium to wondering
what death feels like.

Small-town doctor says they don't have the meds I need
but they do a blood test anyway
so that the results might be in sooner.
Soon enough, I'm in on a stretcher
in an ambulance on a highway watching
the swiss scenery go by
out the back window there's not a lot of traffic.
Maman is scared but relieved
that the travel insurance is taking care of the bill.
I spend a night or two in Lausanne's
high-tech university hospital
there's WiFi so really I'm decently happy.
The nurse takes my electronic music
recommendations before I check out
I'm well enough to get on a plane so we fly back to Ottawa
and to this day we do not know what I caught in the mountains.

Spring 2017

Dreamt I'm strutting across the lobby of a hotel where I work retail,
pass the co-working space the bar the pool table and push aside
the hardwood door to one of the binary water closets.
Find the room padded with sweltering black velvet walls floor ceiling
all black all soft
I begin to melt as I walk forward in a vain attempt
    to relieve myself in black porcelain
but instead I woke up to find my bed soaked in sweat.
I take my temperature for the second time that night — 38.6C.
I tried to keep the temp. down with acetaminophen
but I only delayed the inevitable.

It's 2am, I gather up my necessities and take the night-bus south
to l'Hôpital Notre-Dame because I'm too broke for a cab
Maman is in another country for a conference.
Calmly waltz into the ER take a number wait my turn, they've got my file.
Earlier that night I tried to lie to myself like
oh im just dehydrated i shouldn't have had that last beer
but I felt fever's omens before going to bed.
First few years at conc-University basically each did the same thing to me
I overworked underslept and ignored my body's desire for rest
until it was time to check in as a patient.
Whisked through admissions they've got me in a bed
an IV drip of broad-spectrum antibiotics and saline
to keep me hydrated although No, we don't know what I've caught.
Whatever, fine, do a blood test a blood culture try to figure it out
    if it matters.
I'm there a couple of days.

Back home, we burned your feet by spilling scalding golden tea that
 Maman had just handed over.
She'd gotten back that day from a trip abroad, a conference in Vegas,
and I'd gotten home that day from hospitalization,
a couple of days at Notre-Dame.
That was the month I first read Sontag On Photography
as well as the time my partner was mistaken for my sibling at bedside.
It was the summer I decided to try shooting film
and I still haven't developed all the rolls.
I actually ended up burning the undeveloped rolls.
It's the time, the only time, I asked the nurse if I could snapshot the IV
 being needled in.
So I'd just gotten home and Maman as well, from different journeys.
Scalding flesh with water I tore off the jeans I was wearing (I still wear that
 pair)
and sat on the bed, looking up the right course of action on wikihow.
Soaked my feet in lukewarm water but realized pretty fast
as the bubbles formed on skin
that a doctor should probably have a look at this
so maman helped me stumble to her car and we drove back to the hospital
I had walked home from earlier the same day through MTL
verdant spring holding hands feeling lively and fucking my friend
who was leaving for Toronto that afternoon.
In the interval between sex and getting burned
I finished Sontag and decided to keep taking pictures
because that seemed like a worthy endeavour.

Back at the ER the nice doctor prescribes me morphine
but I smoke tea instead.
Platelet counts way too low, time to take a month off work
defer some exams and visit some family.
Platelets, for the uninitiated reader,
are a component of blood generated in bone marrow
that serve to clot blood and heal wounds.

In other words:
lacking platelets, we bleed.

Sharing Air
2020-05-05

In the midst of pandemic
I have gone on some walks, sat in some municipal parks.
Other people breathe nearby. I wonder where they've been recently.
How many of them bring a hospital's airspace with them to the park?
Just out of the allotted physical range,
I'm aware that they are also breathing.
They talk and laugh and drink and smoke sometimes
making the wind visible for a moment,
inhale and exhale with the world atmosphere.
Wind catches my pores
carries my body dust along with each of yours
so we conspire regardless of distance,
bridging vast expanses across nothingness
in order to be together.

I live very far from the front lines.
I don't know what it's like to live with combat nearby.
All I know of such places has come to me through images videos words,
most of my senses are spared the ample truth: the smells, the shock.
I know only a fantasy, fictitious war.
Yet war and I share an atmosphere.
We breathe within one another.
My breath whispers: How simple, inhale exhale over again
    the first to last thing we'll ever do.
It's the repetition that counts, one breath is nothing for the body, we need air uncounted yet we account for a chemical regime, a specialized diet of far more than oxygen which is poison anyway in overdose. The air we share is a floating, transparent pharmacy not-so-carefully calibrated, and precisely weaponized.

Please welcome the medics wherever there is fighting.

What is there to gain from the veritable assault on human sensory capacity, from mass death? I desire counter-offensive measures, but who doesn't? Anyone whose ever been hurt has tried retaliation, tried hurting back. Lately my reading has taken me into potential histories where men still wreak havoc, but others resist.

The air we share is risky, so we determine how much risk we're willing to handle at a given moment. I conspire to emit air which filters out suffering and positively impact any brief encounter. I share the results with the inevitable passersby no matter which precautions we take. I wear a mask in public indoors and in close quarters but have given up on masking myself for a stroll to the park.

My body is trying its best with what it knows of the long-winded lie that is that there is self and there is other. I trust the precautions I am taking are enough for me and those I interact with. I trust the air with my immune system. But I do not trust my body to visit a hospital right now. I am angry that it has to be this way, and I am scared. I do not know what happens to my body when the numbers stop determining how it exists, but I do not want to measure the passing of time with numbers and test results.

My partner brings their world to me and we share stories whispering back and forth of then there here now conspiring liquid atmospheric coalitions brewing. Limbo feels longer and shorter every single day. Breathing is a reminder of life as well as a way of giving thanks. Over facebook messenger I ask my estranged father what worries him right now. How many people will die, are dying, he says.

I choose to continue sharing air. Circumstances may make that difficult or impossible. I choose this consciously, so I do not bow before inevitability. The inevitable does not rule me. Why should it? I treat those inevitabilities I have learned as parts of the air and blood streams.

Touch screams, loud, when the body feels unknown skin. Brushed up against a cashier's hand as they hand me a receipt, their mouth beyond the counter's plastic shielding. Our breaths shouldn't mingle,

I'm wearing a mask and hopefully they are too. Surface boundaries are tricky. Skin keeps the blood in, but it doesn't keep the world out. Atunement to lived bodies has shifted.

AUTO-IMMUNE HERESY

Stating the obvious helps me stay grounded I guess,
I think it's because I'm used to my life-force being a numbers game.
You know, like stats in an RPG.
Trying to min-max numbers to attain optimal efficiency.
We're basically machines anyway right
like, so many dudes have said that
seems ridiculous though idk.
I think we're more like mycelia
or maybe trees.

A Little Golden Cat
2020-05-13

Mae slides by and I sense the displaced air,
a noticeable shift in housebound stillness.
I do nothing but breathe and pick up the
charge of 2 human bodies
amidst home appliances and neighbours hidden away by walls.

I'm lucky when I discern her specific scent from the others,
when my sense of smell isn't distracted by some noise.
If the fridge hums I can't make her out.
Above the stove there's one of those golden plastic cats
whose arm waves metronomically
with a little solar cell panel.
A plastic Maneki-neko souvenir trinket.
A seated cat, a bib around its neck, a bell or two,
a bastardized Japanese koban coin, a paw raised.

Literally a "beckoning cat," the swinging arm's
tick-tacks are always audible,
like a clock that announces no time in particular when I deign to look over
but rather speaks only to its own presence
   on that stove here in so-called montreal.
I don't know whether the cat ever stops beckoning a timeless now.
All it seems to accomplish is a reminder
   that the old stove's analog time-set is dysfunctional.

The iconic beckoning cat appears to have originated
in the late Edo period, feudal Japan,
and can now be acquired wholesale on Alibaba at the astonishing rate
of up to five-hundred-thousand units per month, shipped out of Xiamen,
a city in the southeastern China beside the Taiwan Strait.
The Maneki-neko in this apartment was manufactured in China,
passed quality control and imported to America,
so say the embossments and sticker on the bottom,
before being purchased and turned into a souvenir in this home.

There are 2 screws in the base that let me take it apart
so I do, in the hopes that peering into the lucky cat's innards will reveal
something essential about the nature of time itself.
What I find instead of a hollow metaphor
is another series of plastic and metal components that come together
to make up the swinging arm mechanism.

Likely harvested anywhere on earth, mined out of deep
time's accretion in the dirt and forged
out of globalized myth—the golden cat is storied.
The Maneki-neko is a symbol of good fortune,
arising out of a story involving a destitute shop/temple/inn;
the poor proprietors take in a hungry and neglected cat.
After being cared for and loved, the cat ventures out front,
sits there and beckons to passers-by,
thus shifting the fortunes of the establishment and bringing prosperity.

Whose idea was this cultural export?
Did they grow up with their own cherished cats either animate or carved?
Either way they turned around and sold
myth down the river for capital gain
because it seemed the logical thing to do.

I don't blame them but that doesn't stop me
from despising the swinging arm
sometimes when I'm just breathing but then
its tack tick tack tick sticks
to my eardrum and I can't shake off
this little cat's little hand.

I mention to Mae that I'm writing about this cat and learn
apparently she bought it years ago in NYC chinatown
when roaming the streets as tourists with friends.
One of them was leading the group astray
everyone was frustrated but ultimately souvenirs were purchased,
packed up in suitcases, brought back to NB
and eventually moved to MTL.
So the cat is here, from everywhere, signalling no time at all.

Sometimes when I'm lucky I lose my sense of object permanence.
Out of willful forgetfulness comes a void full of nothing from which to
    learn.
Things fade in and out of thingness and cease their clutter.
For a time I get to forget what surrounds me, some of it,
breathe as if I weren't aware that the objects that inhabit my day-to-day
are fragments displaced from the earth entire.

Sympathie Sanguine
2020-05-31

BLOODINESS IS A MAGNETISM, an earthiness.
Observing my own arms the veins are hills and tunnels. They bulge and recess in turn. It's commonplace for a nurse in a talkative mood to comment on their quality.
Expert appraisal has it: my veins are ripe for harvest.
Not that any of us are too eager.
Nurses are labouring, sticking needles into veins
for days on end.
Most nurses are highly skilled at this task.
It barely hurts. Commendable.

I'm trying to imagine my own blood.
Create chances to hear it.
Remembering follows loss, memory is split fragments
reassembled in a whole different reality.
Blood is a form of gravity.
I'll go back to the beginning.

The first blood test I remember came soon after blind gain.

I was 5 years old at British Columbia Children's hospital.
The blood draw clinic was a couple floors up from the hospital lobby.
The lobby had this massive plastic tree in it. Like 3 stories tall.
We took the elevator up and upon exit there were a series of signs to follow.

    All the walls on this level were painted sky blue
    and decorated with flying creatures, bears in aeroplanes,
    clouds rainbows sunshine you know, the usual hospital festivity.

So we follow the party to the clinic.
Waiting room was pretty small, maybe 40 chairs.

Blue walls. A TV somewhere in the corner.
Pulp magazines for parents to pretend-read.
Toys laid out on a table.

Arrival and check-in, a little window in the wall
next to a door through which we'd soon pass.

We, being myself, Maman,
the other kids and parents waiting.
The first time, I just sat there
not cognizant of what was about to happen.

My feet didn't reach the floor
maybe my legs were too short or the chair's too long.
Swung back-forth in ignorant anticipation or maybe simple boredom.
Waiting rooms used to elicit boredom for me.
I probably stared at the television,
the best way to forget a body before smartphones.
I've noticed that most hospital waiting rooms
don't have TV shows on anymore.
And they don't call people out by name.

Maybe in the children's hospitals they still do.

At the CHUM the teevees just have numbers on them
and every time the numbers change there's a Ding
so everyone looks up
only to dash the patient hopes of all
except one bored soul whose turn it finally is.

Anyway at BC children's in 2001
they called me by name and we passed into the back room,
through a doorway, and then another,
each room lined with stations
having all the fixings needed for sanitary
blood sample harvest.
I'm led to the deepest section
of blue-walled-room and sat in a too-big LUMEX
designed for maximum clinical comfort.
It dawns on me why we're here.
While the nurse explains the procedure,
I scream.

Before blood was medicine it was earth
born of generations sowing their seeds.
For all the talk of purity,
co-mingling is the way of the world.
Assume that blood itself exists in superposition
and that blood is the locus of spirit.
A mode of transition, transportation,
transmission, diffraction.
In the dirt, blood learns what comes of experimentation.

According to Hebrew scripture,
the very life of the creature is in the blood.

Un flot vivant cette boueuse rivière rouge pleine d'esprit.
Cela serait une grave erreur de penser que les histoires que chuchotent le sang sont sans conflits. Le sang de la mère française-anglaise, du soi-disant Québec, porte des siècles de vie coloniale, cette violence. Par le sang du père Israélien juif d'ascendance Ashkenazi, la souffrance du peuple découle. Et pourtant par hasard me voici.

Some things should be red.
Crimson red, hemochrome.
So red you can not look away.
Blood is variously red based on its level of oxygenation.

Too concerned with the red of blood.
What of its blues?
Result of how light traverses skin on a pale body,
crimson arteries appear blue-green on the surface.

If blood yields knowledge then it also lies.
Barren, the land presided upon by supposed victors
for whom spilt crimson is better than drunk.
Would that the ground forget what flows unto the roots,
yet the fruit remembers torn flesh.

I am no apple picker, but a worm
feeding on the spoils of war.
Bone begets bone and we twirl ever onward,
quick to forget and slow to unlearn.

AUTO-IMMUNE HERESY

Fragmentary days whisper:
the night is not for you to explore.
What is hidden in the blood?

Why must the corpse be boxed or burned,
its water wrought, never free to return?
Upon death, leave me in the earth
or the sea with nothing but a silver ring.
Pine coffins suffocate where decay may pine for roots.
Barriers sunk needlessly, why
individualize even decomposition?
If the law should get in the way,
or the forest be too sparse,
burn the body and scatter ashes amongst the lichen.

A deepened sense of presence on earth inhabits me.
Water, dirt. I am slowing down. Trying to connect
each morning with hunger rather than immediately eating.
Each day is one of heartbreak, healing, and love.
My longing is to know my body, keep it for a while,
and know the place I am going to decompose before decomposing.
Get to befriending the trees there, help the forest heal too.

Years ago, my connection to the earth was ripped away by hospitalization.
Hospitals reared me as a pathological child,
Now my doctor wants to see my blood within a month.
Poison and cure, the body's water is pharma's locus, the bloodstream is why
    and how we get off.

Living blind within sickness,
    I used to trust wholly in medicine's optics and chemistry.
I was afraid of different things before.
    Knew less, and slowly awakened to death.

I can't imagine how the nurse's hands are going to feel,
being the second human's touch since march.

What's happened?
(Slavery Shoah Monotheism Europe Colonies Ecocide)
Nothing, I'm fine.
People say climate change, like change is so bad.
Octavia Butler taught me God is change,
as inevitable as love, life itself.
The whole cycle of infinitesimal parts
together making matter and ether.

Why make a bloodbath of living?
Is it out of fear that after-life is being withheld?
Yet change is very much alive,
in all its bloodiness and its disease.
Here's how I feel lately: Civilization is not an inevitability.
It is an idea, humanity's attempt at self-definition by fragmentation.
Humanity's prayer to death.

No one has ever told me I am going to die of an illness.
Not before, not now. My doctor said:

> "The odds of you dying to covid are near zero.
> I know you won't do anything reckless."

He told me so over the phone.
Fair enough, haematology has kept me alive thus far.

In dreams I don't see the blood drawing happen
only empty blue hallways and the echos of my wailing.
Now it seems that was the moment my own mortality first mattered.
What do you think children in cities feel right now?
I don't know, probably they are afraid,
they may be afraid of death, I don't know.
I loved being a child, call it whatever you want.
People don't get that freedom long at all.

Longing for Heat
2020-07-21

HEAT OFF LIPS PINK
And engorged all day
Mouths back and forth
tasting skin in heat
The humidex first hit
40 this year today.
After dinner we sprawl
red couch
redhead red cunt
and I, drink
kombucha, vodka
water with lemon
skin soft despite
sweat and besides
we choose closeness
sticky as it is.
The AC isn't installed
because neither of us
likes the dry air
so I'll see how long
I can be warm.
The heat is like this
every summer and
every summer the
heat gets worse
The clit's beauty
My index soft
then hard
basking.

Bright blue broken pixels
lack info against eyelids
Lefteye hyperactive
hardly leaves me be.
Turns out
The words are real,
the jobs ain't.

   Who cares, doc?
My dear Dr., do you partake in the blood of Christ?
What about blood magick, doc?
What do you make of that?
How do you like your steaks?
Do you ever go trapping, look a wild animal in the eye
as you slaughter them with a knife?
No, of course not, seeing as you won't bleed me yourself.

Division of wage labour says that you tick boxes on a sheet,
stamp a signature, and look at numbers on a screen
after the nurse has relieved me of blood and the lab tech has scanned it.

How come you didn't decide to be an accountant instead, doc?
Must be because an accountant doesn't get to
chemically re-balance human bodies and see how that turns out.
Must be because an accountant's numbers are fictional abstractions
while your numbers are anchored in blood. Blood money's real too, doc.
Some accountants get to count up the numbers for their boss
whose business it is to bleed people day in day out.
Violence specialists.

Stroke of a pen on a ledger, offshore,
how's that different from a gunshot, doc?
What if my blood were inside black skin instead, doc?
Would the government still pay my bills?
Maybe they would, just to see
that sixty thousand dollars a year go to
a multinational pharmaceutical company
instead of social welfare.

The Oncology Ward In The Sky
2020-08-25

Biking west along side roads,
I whiffed the hospital complex two blocks away,
industrial cleanser seeps through the black cotton mask.
Lock up, walk the final 100 feet.

First, disinfect hands.
People cluster in an attempt to form a line and
follow the signposted instructions.
We're all masked. Security guards mill about,
a nondescript hospital employee guides people where they need to go.

> *Do you have an appointment? Where are you headed?*

Centre Intégré de Cancérologie, 14th floor,
I've got a blood test today.

> *Oh, you know you have a separate entrance and elevators right?*
> *Here, this way, come with me.*
> *By coming in through there, you won't have to wander*
> *the entire hospital or touch stuff that's "disinfected"*
> *though no one really cleans it.*

Thank you, I say, and ponder the horror of that last statement as I disinfect my hands again though I haven't touched anything and make my way to the Oncology-Elevators. Two of us are whisked up in a socially-distanced elevator ride. Maximum occupancy of 4, one person per floor-sticker.

Upstairs I am greeted by a nurse who asks the usual symptom-probes.
The nurse's right hand brushes up against my palms as she leans in
to spray sanitizer and disinfect me once more.
I didn't even press the elevator buttons.
A volunteer in a polka-dot bow-tie
walks me down the long waiting room
to point out the blood work reception desk,
which has not moved in the 6 months since I was last here.
I was supposed to return sooner, of course.

- They've been working on adding a third even taller wing to the CHUM. In the waiting room I always look down at the progress. Almost done now. Not just another hole in the ground.
- I used to get my blood tests done at Notre-Dame, an old old hospital on Sherbrooke, opened in 1880. The CHUM, built in 2017, has another high capacity blood-draw clinic on the main floor of D-wing, but I've never sat there in that glass box within the heart of the skyscraper complex with no view outside for patients. For some reason I take the elevator to Oncology.
- Once though I stayed overnight at the Nouveau-CHUM in an ER hallway on a cot under fluorescents. It was mid-march of 2019. I sat in receptive silence, half-lotus, eyes closed, listening, not sleeping. Notice, the overworked nurses are torn between the desire to provide comfort and the expectation of staying back, respecting the distance imposed by pain, by sickness. How does it feel to have disease constantly on your mind? Every conversation I've had in the past week has either been about illness or violence.
- In the morning my managing haematologist was on duty and came to see me at bedside.

I said I'm fine.
He said
You're not fine listen to these numbers.
We'll up your dose of Revolade
Deliver intravenous iron
and Request an appointment with the gastroenterologist
because surely if you're this anaemic your stomach must be bleeding.

Alright then, I guess.

AUTO-IMMUNE HERESY

As he discharges me, the doctor jokes
about how nice the rooms are up on the 15th floor,
as if hospitalization is the right thing to chuckle warmly about.
I think he's well-intentioned and has a good grasp of haematological
medicine but I was glad to leave, go home,
and spend a month in bed resting
while the weather turned warm.
Out the 14th floor waiting-room window I see the sky, the city, beyond.
Nearby another patient sits down and opens a book:
The Most Beautiful Quebecois Poems.

I glance back outside
a small brown-speckled spider weaves its web
across the glass. From where I'm standing
it's bigger than the construction workers,
bigger than the pedestrians, almost the size of the police cruiser
two intersections away. Waiting there,
refusing to sit in the disinfected chairs,
I wonder what good all the poetry in the world
will do this single arachnid
spinning its home over Mooniyang.

The centre de prélèvements is a resolutely hygienic space.
Blood draws occur 7am-3pm M-F.
Wait times are short for patients who get blood taken here up high.
I ask a nurse how many blood tests a day she's doing lately.
It depends, but a little over 100.

We're checking my auto-immune system,
it's been known to eat away at me.
Platelets, also called thrombocytes,
are tiny cells that are essential for normal blood clotting.
When platelets are particularly low,
internal bleeding is a risk,
and I get acutely aware of my skin's surfaces
its folds, distracted by specks of the outer world
that brush up against it, egg-albumin thin.
The circulatory system is a series of veinous corridors,
highways, canals, transit arteries carrying blood along.
The lightest pressure might bruise and the lightest scrape might tear.
So we test.
Sharp metal insertion somewhere along the arm. Middling.

Primary symptoms are: excessive bruising, bruising in excess of what one would've expected for the amount of trauma, or bruises that are totally unexplained.

When my daily life is asymptomatic, the blood work makes sure to rectify the notion that everything is normal. Platelet counts outside the norm have been my everyday for 19 years. I wonder whether we'll get to stop counting anytime soon?

Internal bleeding's a slow dissolving of veinous layers melding into a contiguous ocean of blood. Carefully mapped out roads falling into disarray as in-betweens flood. Microscopic terror as a shortage of platelets leads to tidal waves overcoming the sea walls under maintained, decimated by an overzealous team of white blood cells.

If this shows up to the naked eye at all, it's usually as 'petechiae'; tiny red pinpoints in the skin, little red-blue dots along the arms, the legs, around the groin. Mini-bruises.

Even invisible illness is subject to sight. Can we stop counting anytime soon? Put blood under a microscope and find out just how its balance turns out. Break it down into categories for testing, count out with frightening exactitude just how much of this that and whatever else my body happened to contain at 7:32am on August 25th, 2020.

My haematologist's job is precisely to make sense of the clinical minutiae contained within blood. Logic takes a crack at making sense of our lifeblood, and I can't help but laugh.

It's time I got out of here.

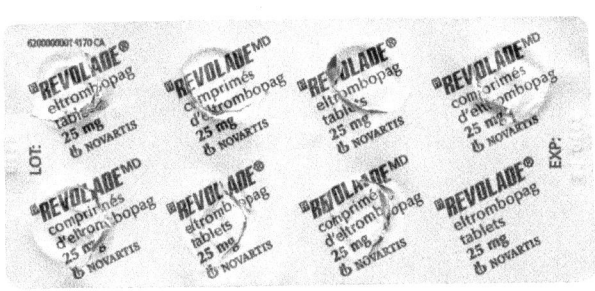

Patience

Sainte-Anne-des-Monts
2020-11-11

Où patientons-nous?
   l'aéroport
   en file d'attente
   pour le courrier
   pour que l'eau se mette à bouillonner
   lorsque le four se réchauffe
   et à l'hôpital

Le lit d'hôpital: lieu du patient; espace rituel; espace professionnel; intime; transportatif; hétérotopique; contemplatif; l'espace de la vie de la fin.
Du lit, les patient.es observent l'action logistique d'un support vital humain et machinique. Le corps patient, au lit, évolue, se transforme au fur et à mesure que la médecine complète son travail.

Comment faire la métaphysique du patient?
Lentement.

Patiente est celle qui attend l'heure de son départ.
"Quand pourrai-je partir?"
La patiente ne peut pas savoir combien de temps durera sa situation.
Entre deux, comment s'occupe-t-elle?
Pourquoi attendre?
Qu'est-ce qui l'empêche de partir?
Qu'est-ce que la souveraineté corporelle?

Le corps au lit – D'abord, il n'y a pas toujours une horloge.
Ou bien les yeux ne fonctionnent pas, et on est pas encore habitué alors c'est une grosse désorientation. Mais peu importe l'heure, c'est les autres qui s'en occupent. Pour le lit la seule préoccupation c'est l'attente. Rien de mieux pour se remettre que l'immense Rien du lit perpétuel. Ce n'est pas à ce corps de se mêler de ces affaires. Assise couchée deux oreillers ou bien trois, les couvertures bien blanches question d'apercevoir la saleté. Autour du lit il y a des rideaux, des gadgets. Au moins une machine qui fait Beep, Beep, mais probablement plus d'une. Acier inoxydable le lit avec ses barrières amovibles et ses roues qui permettent l'examination sous tout plein d'angles.
L'aiguille me réveilla tous les jours. Je fixais dans les yeux celleux qui me piquèrent. Je prenais plaisir à démontrer ma compréhension, bien que mon corps n'ait pas encore appris à faire usage de sa boîte vocale. Un autre joyau pour la science médicale. Synthétisons la cybernétique en sang, disaient-ils. Et pourquoi-donc? Ai-je demandé de naître? Chacune de mes vies commence au bras gauche. Doucement, doucement le coulis y entre par le portail où se fraie l'aiguille. Métallique cylindre qui nous rapproche, vous et moi. L'aiguille me réveilla tous les jours. J'existe dans les yeux de celleux qui me piquèrent. Je prends plaisir.
Puis les yeux s'ouvrent, et l'infirmière affirme que le traitement est fini pour la journée. Ce corps que je vis dans le présent achève son assimilation de la force vitale que portent les autres sangs. Dommage.
Qu'est ce que la patience? Vertu
Patienter? acte

La patience c'est l'attente certaine d'avoir une fin, sans savoir ce que cette fin réserve ni quand elle arrivera.

C'est un choix constant que d'abandonner la certitude, la confiance. Nul doute plus simple d'accepter ce qui se dit ici et là sans trop douter. Peut-être qu'on se rassoit, bien confortable, sur le divan, visionnant la télé, l'écoute plus ou moins attentive. Suffit de ne pas questionner, le programme se fait par soi-même. Plaisant? Non, car le monde largement dépeint n'est pas plaisant. Mais simplifié, alors réconfortant.

La patience c'est l'attente certaine d'avoir une fin,
sans savoir ce que cette fin réserve ni quand elle arrivera.
Attendre:
- la mort
- le résultat
- les diagnostics
- la pluie et le beau temps
- le jour du jugement dernier
- le levain
- la mijoteuse
- le coucher du soleil et la levée de la nuit
- Godot
- un appel, un rappel

You understand how frustrated I am, surely?
No child ought to be told who or what they are.
But of course, most are.
This then is a call to preach heresy,
to deny all imposed identities,
and define by reinvention.

June 2015-Nov 2020: the pills got me through school.

They imposed stability and raised the baseline.
But when I'd get elsewise sick,
I still needed IVIG, or iron,
or perhaps just rest.

Doctors never told me to rest.
I was young and young folks should be out
taking on the world!

But what if auto-immunity demands a life of quietude?
What if I'll never be a mountain biker or ultramarathon runner
or capital A Athlete with the physique of a greek god/dess?

All the treatment I ever received was not designed
to heal or remove illness,
but just treat symptoms.
But what if symptoms are just the body demanding rest?

Thrombocytopenia leaves me at risk of bleeding;
not in itself a fatal disease.
Life is a risk regardless.

My body is auto-immune.
Immunity is unique to each body.
There's no treatment plan which removes the potential for bleeding.

To bleed is to live.
The only knowledge I'm relying on now
is embodied knowledge.
Of how I feel and what I sense on a daily basis.

I am writing my body anew,
tending to its stories and finding the past
is stranger than the documents imply.

It's November now. Pandemic, still.
I stifle the urge to check provincial infection numbers
and download books instead.

My computer has recently become a much friendlier device.
I got a screen that doesn't hurt my eyes.
It's turning into a desktop-book, just like I always dreamed.

No meandering the internet without a purpose,
all the content I consume is by choice.
This, too, is making a body.

Willfully forgetting the past in order to move forward.
What we're doing is shaking off trauma like a wounded deer,
   spasmodically.
Matter of doing rather than merely observing flesh's reactivity. Taking stock of bodily anxieties to integrate and loosen the tensions that have stacked subconsciously over years of life. Sitting meditation is not enough on its own to dislodge the stone of sense-memory in your chest. Stone which holds a past as yet unknown to our waking mind. Sitting may reveal some of your story, doubtful whether a clear flow will be made to pass only by bringing attention to the spot. Maybe with many months and years. Meditation must not be undertaken with an end goal. Circling some imaginary end turns the practice into a chore rather than a steady devotion. Not unlike caring for and maintaining friendships.

You are my dearest friend and my most intimate lover.
You carry us throughout it all, the joy of dance
the pain of needles
and still you embrace life anew each breath.
Thank you.

I used to strive for a return to a mythical healthy Before,
but in fact moving forward in resolving my bodily enigma means
integrating the old into a process of aging
into a body that's never existed before.

Years ago you were deemed by some men
in labcoats to be somehow wrong.
How long we believed them and their numbers.
To them you are subject to categorical classification like
boy/sick/anemic/thrombocytopenic.
Ha!

I remember lying in bed desperately running my hands over your neck your neck your skull seeking a pulse anywhere. So long as fingers found the thump thump it meant you were still alive. When I couldn't find any I'd go sleep with Maman because her life force would save you, surely.
The heartbeat found in so many crooks and crannies where your veins surface was the only assurance I had that you were still there anchoring me, keeping me grounded rather than floating lost in the cosmos behind your eyelids.
Your fingertips were the access point for sensation, the means I had for connecting through touch long before we learned the words proprio- or intero-ception. Developing a vocabulary for your capacities has the stunning effect of producing new possibilities for existing.

I feel perfectly at home within you.
This was not always the case.
For years sensation was a necessary evil
I tried by every means to minimize.

Revolade imposes stress on the body.
Tension build-up as chemical release creates reactions.
I feel tightness that begins in my eyes and needles red to the base of my skull.
I am taking 75mg a day as of writing this line (Oct 26 2020).
That's 50+25mg each morning, after breakfast.
C'est dans la moelle, osseuse tant qu'épinière, que je ressens la chimie médicale.
Revolade is: Eltrombopag olamine thrombopoetin receptor agonist

Meds oct 26 around 7am.
Rush of anxiety at 1pm.

Earlier today my stoole was of solid soft texture and medium brown,
held together well in 3 small logs.
Water had a red tint.
Beets last eaten 2 days ago, I think?
Meals yesterday: oats, pizza, bean chili.
Can black beans change stool color?
Cooked from dry myself.
No stomach aches but anxiety held onto that red tinge--
fear of blood.
(it was because of pickled beets)

Meds
oct 27-28-29 : 50mg @ 8am.
30th, 50mg 9am
31st 50mg 830am
Nov 1 same
nov 2 same
nov 3 11am

Death is a sculptor. Decay a sublime performance.
Yet obscene, shunned, relegated to other spaces, inaccessible
a matter for experts and numbers, not for friends.
Who among us does not obsess?
I must unlearn so much.

I want to avoid banal and obvious generalizations such as: what I eat matters.
(Platelet helpers: Folates, B9, B12, vit. C (raw), vit. D, vit. K, Iron)
It is a matter of being patient there with/in the organism.
I am the golem and the druid both.
Locating the philosophy and practice of healing oneself with/in blood.
La sang la moelle la peau les os les intestins.

What are the sensory receptors which detect chemicals in blood? When were thrombocytes discovered? By what other names is this clotting agent known? Where are the stories of staunched bleeding?

Je m'oppose à quelconque véridiction de corporéalité. Chaque corps s'auto-compose. Les corps sont des phrases musicales, de mouvement, de pensée, de désir. Les corps humains se partagent certains détails, c'est pourquoi nous sommes une espèce.

On November 11th, 2020,
I stopped taking my meds for the first time,
unsupervised. It sort of worked.

Taking Back My Body
2020-12-21

AUTO-IMMUNITY IS A CALL to attend to one's inner life.
It is my body signifying without language,
in a grammar unique to my physiology,
that attention must be turned inward.

There is no goal, only process.
Learning a sensory lyric leads ever deeper into itself,
and isn't that enough? Insight contains in its
two syllables the entire experience.
My body is made in the process of encounters.

Auto-immunity is far removed from the alleged
self-destructive resistance of a biological system gone haywire.
Not pathology, but compassion for a body, bodies,
that are unbounded from the physical contraint of materialism.

Soma is the teacher along the path of self-compassion.
Not a battleground. Not a machine. Not code. Not optional.
Perhaps the only thing which is not optional:
one's own flesh, sensation, and accompanying psyche.
Once alive, that is all there is.

Yet how much effort did I expend to forget? To escape?
To ignore the impulses with which you communicate with me?
I am sorry. I wish I'd listened sooner.
At least my attention is devoted to you now.

Blood flows for knowledge.
One must bleed, have bled, to seek.
Who said autoimmunity is a dysfunction?
Isn't menstruation a form of autoimmunity?
Then again, pharmacology removes such bleeding as well.
All the body's bleeding, it seems, must be carefully managed,
regulated rather than left to spontaneity.
Control over blood is control over life.

I shed concerns about the facts
of body blood and autoimmunity.
I am concerned solely with my first-person experience,
my own apprehension of flesh.

A month has gone since I stopped my medication.
This morning upon waking my sheets
had left many smudges of red on my skin.
I noticed in the shower.
I told myself perhaps the pinpoint bruises
are from the heavy straps of the grocery bags.

Some petichia are apparent on my upper body, biceps, chest.
My stomach has goosebumps. Either from fear or cold.
Anxiety gathers like black foam around my liver.
Tension in my gut as I wonder whether to eat,
wonder what to eat. Few things are appetizing.
I'm craving more meat, far less sugar.

I gave up one upside (reliable platelet counts)
with many potential downsides.
In exchange for a downside
(the return of thrombocytopenia),
with many potential upsides.

Dec 18 2020: Petichia appear on hands+wrists,
especially left side, around 5pm.
Looking down at my hand and discovering it covered with bruises
brought a rush of anxiety bubbling up my spine
into an explosion of brain fog.
Noise, monochromatic, crowding all sensation.
Light-headed I lay down and discover my body is not in any pain.
Fear is mental, with physical effects.
Symptoms nearly gone by 7pm.

Morning Dec 19th: symptoms gone.

The process of healing is anything but linear.
No teleology of worse to better to best.
Only sickness, in waves.
Sitting with that.
Feeling its variety.
Autoimmunity is perhaps a harsh teacher.
Its lessons are written in blood upon the moist parchment.

Autoimmunity is perpetual.
The body is the nexus through which time is enacted in space.
Cyclical returns defy linear narratives of healing
premised on empire's prescriptive timeline
of how a human life may be lived.
Some see the body as static, preformed,
pre-determined biotechno-processes.
Autoimmunity defies such simplistic reductionism.

Is this an exit?
I did not tell the medical staff I ceased my treatment.

I look up from my phone
with the urge to plunge into a search for escape.
   Duckduckgo: "Monasteries in Canada"
But it is not so simple to heal.

I am where I am, here, and I know I am staying put.
The weight of place and the weight of self.
Commitment to new patterns exposes the rhythmic
   tides of solitary doubt.
What am I so angry about? Why am I so confused?
The isolation is crushing, mulching.
I feel like I'm composting my whole lived experience
   and it is infuriatingly slow.
I feel like nothing is leading anywhere.
   LIMBO drags ever onward and back.

The body sweats out the chemistry and I
stop costing the province 4500$/month.
The molecular coercion keeping my stem
cells constantly productive fades away,
and the truth of a body in mourning is allowed to reappear.

My grief is visible in the bruise
that takes two weeks to heal.
It is visible in the petechiae
that constellate my arms, thighs, feet.
Notice grief when I shit
and the t.p comes away splotched with fresh blood.

How do I live in a way that is not self-destructive,
not harmful to life, and reconcile that with grieving?
Why am I bleeding? What did I do?

Communion
2021-01-207

How do I communicate with the invisible aspects of my body,
with that which is occulted?

The occulted body is literally that which is the body unseen.
Kinaesthetic awareness. Motorsensory education. Somatic experience.
Blood and tissue and all we ingest. Digestion is occult.

Inner alchemy, breath, the shifting locus of intentional focus.
Sensing blood and tissue and bone, the watery and the earthen self.
There's no quantitative analysis available
for making rational sense of this relationship,
there is only a quality of divine apprehension
that may be glimpsed when I am allowed to return to the source.

Void of preconceived notions limiting what may be possible,
I encounter a depth charge that shatters expectations.
Taking the heart for a drum beat, beat, beat
   ever onward inward seeking not after answers
   but for ever more precise questions.
For it is in the asking that insight is revealed.

I pause, and wonder whether this journey is plausible.
Balk at myself momentarily: "Ha! You're in no position to understand."
   Yet shed these doubts, for if not I then whom?
Surely no external measure no number holds the key to my flesh.
It is not written in law that I may not know myself.
Any such contract is none that I have agreed to, and as such is one I reject.
   No intermediary may intervene on my behalf,
   no priest/ess teach me what is true.

The needle interjects:
I shall enumerate the reality of your blood.
Only if I should let it.

Again today I sat in a blue chair to bleed red
feed the sterile machinery. To what end?

Months without testing have left me alive,
awake to internal life.

A nurse asks: "Who told you to do that?"
No one, it was an autonomous decision.

We'll see what the doctor has to say about the numbers
abstracting my lifeblood, when we next speak on the phone.

I know myself by practicing, by attempting,
by sharing, by delving, by attending, by devotion.
I seek the questions to illumine the body's
iterative becoming, it's multiplicity of discontinuities.
Never shall I presume to have reached a conclusion.

Never shall the flesh have revealed itself fully.
To make such presumptions is folly
from there the inevitable decline.

So long as I maintain my ignorance,
I have much to learn, so much to learn.

This week really kicked my ass. On a daily basis I whirl between depths and heights of confusion and certainty. I miss doing drugs. 2017-2019 are marked by intermittent cannabis, psilocybin, LSD and DMT use. Seeking spiritual-scientific hyperthick multidimensionality. "Am I doing what I ought to be doing?" always on my mind. The short of it is that there is no "should" or "ought."
Picked up Brothers Karamazov today; Ivan's Grand Inquisitor, with his polemic against the Almighty, and man's inability to handle freedom.
Am I unable to handle freedom? What does freedom mean to me?
   Would I rather have my life dictated to me?
I have been choosing to eat according to auto-immunity for a week, with minor slip-ups.
It's going okay. I called Maman last night to complain that it feels like nothing I do is effectual. She reminds me:
You are undergoing huge transitions.
And so I am.

Here's where I'm at:
I live alone
I don't smoke
I don't drink
I don't watch TV
I don't watch Movies
I don't Follow The News
I don't drink coffee
I don't eat grains
I don't eat legumes
I don't eat sugar.
I sit in contemplation
I read books
I cook for myself
I go on walks
I talk to friends
I visit my grandmother
I sleep
I listen to selected podcasts.

My dreams lately have been about learning, workshopping, being taught
by many teachers. I hear that when the student is ready, the teachers
appear. I believe my mystery school is in my unconscious. There, and
also on the internet, in the texts. I want to live a mystical life, a magical
life, a mysterious life, an enchanted life, a godly life, a daoist life, a natural
life, a simple life, a good life.
And I wonder, what does that mean?

Love and Joy and Sex and Compassion and Strategy and
Ritual and Passages and Thinking and Speaking and
Birthing and Decaying and Growing and Sowing and
Reaping and Listening and Singing and Shouting and
Seeing and Freezing and Heating. No deficiency and
no excess. Always cycling back.

Imperfection reigns here. Amidst confusion, I breathe in out deep as ever
possible but I feel bloated, weighed down by the unknowns. Why is
my body this way? How did it come to be? What can I do? Do the
not-doing, says the Dao. Therein lies a key, for certain. Wu Wei helps
me glean new insight, new possibilities. Ever a quest for such avenues as
yet unexplored.
This way or that? A new path or old? Am I here for myself or for another?
Are we together or apart? I've never ceased exploring, all I can say is that
rational sense is overrated. I don't want your logic, your boxes. But I'm
trying to understand how they work.

Regressing Moves Forward
2021-02-01

9AM, I TAKE 25MG Revolade.
First dose since November.
Yesterday a bruise appeared spontaneously on my right hand ring finger while I walked to Mamie's. I am accepting the efficacy of medicine, I suppose. I am not going to let my body self-destruct while I scramble for alternatives. No, I will instead find safe, stable ground from which to carry on. This decision feels like failure, like admitting defeat.
Auto-immunity tells me the world is toxic, the body rebels, and I must respond in the ways that best assure my quality of life. I am saddened that I must remain in this particular entanglement, with this particular molecule. Why? Why does this remedy bother me? Is it purely the cost? Am I so opposed to medicine or to profit? Have I not been treated well? Why fight?
I want to collaborate with the chemistry activating my bone marrow. Thank you, Pharmacy, for making it possible that a small daily pill lead to the generation of more numerous blood platelets. Indeed, such precision is miraculous and ought not be shunned outright. This return to treatment is not failure, it is a testament to the non-linearity of healing. I now have a simple confirmation and perhaps that is what I sought.
I am still auto-immune. The beauty and chaos of winging it is that ultimately there are no wrong answers. The autonomy of embodied life lies in choosing how to interpret one's relation to the world.

The summer before first grade there was a heatwave in QC City. Maman was looking for a job, for a place to live, for a school. I was going to day-camp. I'd been sick/blind nearly a year. We left Vancouver to be closer to family, to save money. First week of camp I got up the courage to stay overnight with the other kids. First day of first grade I didn't go to school because Maman couldn't bring me. Instead my sitter, some college student, asked me what I wanted to do that day. Movies or museums? Easy choice, museums. The oldest colonial city on Turtle Island has excellently stocked imperial showrooms, no doubt.

It is not that the sick child is not talked about, or even invisible.
We have our own hospitals, TV spots, fundraisers.
Rather the sick child is monstrous, abhorrent, pitiable.
The sick child is voiceless. A body to whom things happen;
unfortunate, sad, oh-im-so-sorry things.
The sick child in Canada is an icon.
Always the first victim, the most vulnerable.
The most susceptible to environmental racism and differential governance.

When I got diagnosed, my single mother quit her job
relied on the goodwill of friends.
   We didn't have health insurance anyway.
   Why would we? Canada's got it covered, right?
But so-called "universal healthcare" only applies to certain treatments.
   My mother went into debt to keep her sick child treated.
In The Argonauts, Maggie Nelson's third-party account of their child says Iggy "couldn't care less" at having his body handled by medicine. This is an example of an adulthood shrug, Maggie's ignoring the signification of testing upon a body that will bear the (in)visible marks of illness for its entire life, as many of us do. But Trauma does not preclude joy. Is medical intrusion necessarily, inherently traumatic?
The (chronically, terminally, irreparably) sick child is a poster,
   a footnote, a statistic by which institutions
   seek funding and conduct research.
Iggy is reified as a statistic in Nelson's account
because their mother could not resist the lure
of the exceptional sick child who pulls through despite the odds.
(just like me, dear reader, hurrah)

The sick child is the object of fascination
in countless books, studies, memoirs of parenthood,
sermons and prayers, and many, many oil paintings.

The narrative is almost always the same:
Years of mis-diagnosis, disbelief by doctors,
suffering, as life is turned topsy-turvy
(How *could this happen to us?*)
eventual acceptance
and barely veiled moralizing
about the myth of recovery
(aren't we all sick anyway?)

The parent of the sick child is afraid, so afraid. What worse fate than to hold your child's hand as they whither away, body seemingly turned against itself, unable to walk, a fading living limbo.

Memoirs of sickness (this one included)
are fetishistic at best, romantic doldrums at worst.
Is anyone really interested in our hundreds of E.R visits?
Why? The emergency room is a circle of hell.
It is boring, tiresome, and smells awful.
Like barely preserved decomposition.

A healthy reader picks up an illness memoir to glimpse life in That Other Place, crosses themselves and kisses their healthy child's forehead: "Please God, may such a thing never befall our family." But of course, sickness isn't so easily warded off.
It is not the intention of this text to say: Ignore doctors! Any reading which takes that to be the point is shallow at best. Once, clearly, for the record: Medical practice is at times essential and life-saving.
Nor is this tract a call to internet-search quackery. What is essential is bodily self-knowledge, and an end to total reliance upon the tools of experts with an MD. I am writing to give shape to the fury, and thus cease being merely patient, merely sick.

We never complained of poor treatment.

I wrack my memory now for instances
of incompetence or negligence.
All I can say for my case is that sometimes
a nurse would fail to do their duty with a needle,
and many pinpricks were made where one should have sufficed.

But what is one needling among hundreds?

There are banal instances of bother
common to inpatient life
(getting to the washroom with an IV pump? Annoying.)
but over time one gets habituated quite well.

For some years I felt that it is much preferable
to be in a hospital if one is sick.
Where better?
My logic was that the odds of survival
must be greater in such a place.
Now I'm not always so sure.

The only real complaint I have is the food,
and perhaps that's why
I don't think of hospitalization
as necessarily beneficial, now.

How is anyone supposed to get stronger eating white bread,
corn flakes, mashed potatoes, and juice from concentrate?

But I forget myself, and hear now clearly
the inevitable retort:

Free healthcare though!

Yes indeed,
but how much does the endless IV drip really cost?
It's a matter of method, of priorities, of budgeting.
What contracts underlie the treatment practices
in public institutions?
What long-term commitments to pharmacy?

Auto-immune is itself a word
that would do violence to the wholeness of being,

A rejection of self by self, a biological self-loathing.
Repent! For thy cells do you wrong. I reject this morality.
Auto-immunity is not an individual state of being.

But what better turn of phrase?
I've given up on explanation,
and will content myself with stating:
If I am to heal, it is because I am kind
to the cells that compose me.

How much youth uselessly buried?
Maybe home will be discovered in writing about you.
Raised and medicated near and far from our birthplace,
yet always rootless, treading chlorinated water.
Taking it slow has revealed a hollowness where a spleen used to rest
and in the nodes of a liver recuperating.
What we're doing here is writing up blueprints, cryptic as any other.

Knowing my body is sacred activism.
It once seemed abhorrent in every way.
Monstrous, without divinity.
Years of setting you down on the page,
pages of organs, of shattered conceptions,
of disavowal, of leaning into gravity.
Would that these pages held
reams of philosophical nuance
where instead only fragments of experience are laid bare.

How sick and pitiable some reader may find us.
You, a bloody mess. Me, frantically attempting to make sense of it all.
The modes of address are idiosyncratic at best,
disjointed on average, incomprehensible at worst.
So what? These pages are yours and mine,
shared with the world but never bowing to its demands for propriety.

I'm after is a sort of sanguine seeing.
A blood sight
through which genealogy may be known and harnessed.
What I came to realize is that Revolade occluded the possibility
of knowing the blood that flows through me as my own.
Blood remains ever co-mingled with, well, everything.
(How do the Californian grapes that I am eating change my physiology?)
It is a matter of gaining more minute control over what we absorb.
Voluntary detoxicity where possible.

Foods have subtler impacts than pharmacy but also offer fewer risks.
Leave fewer traces and are (perhaps) less resource intensive to create.
Why exactly is a 28-day course of 75mg Revolade 4500CAD?
Surely the ingredients aren't so cost intensive?
How are global supply chains mobilized
to create thrombopoetin receptor agonists?
Putting these questions down in writing hurts,
in the way confronting any unpleasant unknown may hurt.
Prior to finding factual answers, I can only speculate that what I find
(if indeed such information is traceable)
will reinforce a hatred of vertically integrated exploitation
with new details telling me what I basically already know.
So why hunt? Why seek out the nitty-gritty? Must we?

Sadness and hunger are often confusedly intermingled feelings.
Deep in the gut, clenching tension.
I'll regularly eat when I'm already sated just to quench the feeling.
I've only recently realized this. It's difficult to admit to myself that I am sad.
That the muscular holding impulse is a defence mechanism
I developed to shield me from my feelings.
A tight muscle hides sensation.

My gut acts as a barrier between the upper and lower places of the body.
Right around my centre of gravity at the navel is where tension hides.
Honest feeling reveals that the impulse to eat right after lunch
stems from a fear of digestion.
Both food and emotion require parasympathetic integration.
It's not yet clear, the source of this specific habit.

There are any number of reasons to avoid integrating/digesting negativity.
What I know now is that without making space inwardly for the sorrow to ebb and flow, it will inevitably overrun the territory, as rivers caught behind a dam. Flooding damages so many disparate and interconnected aspects of self/world ecology. Superficial methods for instant gratification (A snack!) bloat the canals of feeling where/when sadness may be felt deeply, as not merely pain, but as an essential marker of enfleshed reality. As above, so below. If I do not allow the body to become hungry, I will not discover what it desires and, by the same token, what it needs.
The thrombopoetin receptor agonist I took for 5 years had the medically palliative effect of (mostly) maintaining my body's platelet counts around the normal range. The drug also comes with a long list of side-effects, chief among which is anaemia. Funny, the doctors were unable to find the source of the anemia detected through blood work, so I took huge iron supplements for three years.
None of us thought to consider ceasing the main pill. Instead, more tests, more pills, more needles. Absurd.
A phone call from the gastroenterologist:
Her voice rings hollow with cavernous surprise
upon learning my body's iron eventually corrected itself
without their pills or needles.
Shy, I suggest the medicine may have been a culprit.
She disagrees, but is pleased
that her needless test
can still make it into the report.

AUTO-IMMUNE HERESY

I am living through a whirlwind right now.
I feel physically renewed,
each day more attuned to needs.
Physically awakening to overwhelming optionality.
Each day assailed with endless What Ifs.
Some acts are underway.
Some future worry seeps into the daily where it needs not.
My dreams are teachers.
The world's inexorable advance continues shifting.
A day contains so much yet so little.
A night so short yet so expansive.
Who said anything about winning and losing?
What about letting go of focus? Practice.
Sometimes I am anxious to get going.
Other times staying put is bliss.
Certain decision are within my control,
and many uncertainties exist without.
Do I seek simple passive comfort? No.
Am I after integrated wellbeing? Surely.

From the well meaning friend
to the polemical witch,
everyone agrees:
One must first heal oneself.

No need to create harsh laws of self-rule.
Such discipline is not only joyless, it is harmful.
Do what is of interest, and nurture ongoing discovery.
Certainly, some things are better avoided,
because we have learned through trial and error
that bone and blood respond poorly to exposure.

This extends into the mediatic.
Don't ingest harmful thoughts needlessly,
and allow time for digesting the emotions that arise from encounters.
We are not in a hurry.
Calls to productivity are best ignored outright. A diagnosis of autoimmunity blames the individual body for shortcomings in the world. Medicine refuses to acknowledge that 24/7 lives of submission to capital are inherently sick demand, and thus turns suffering inward, as though every doctor were Nietzsche diagnosing the Christians. When medicine speaks of auto-immunity it does not mean a body evoking demands to attention. No, the body becomes the enemy.
Well, I refuse.
My body is not my enemy.
It is my lover and teacher and my best friend.
It is the vessel of cosmic life through which I am
    enfleshed, however briefly,
and I will not submit its corporeality to management.

If one's inner experience won't convince others,
then it is best to cease seeking after external validation,
and trust instead inward.
Don't seek for what is already within you.
Rather, accept its presence and behave accordingly.
Evaluating the situation is of course an ongoing effort.
But why collapse time even further by worrying about a future that is
    malleable?
For now, live now. Much is revealed with careful listening to stillness.
I repeat: there is no rush. Rest.

What does fixing do?
It implies brokenness,
as if a given version of self could not harness
the beauty of wellbeing without external influence.

As vultures, we seek for that which serves us in the ruins.
The thing of beauty is discovery of inner experience's malleability.
As much as the world makes me, I make the world.
Why doubt what has yet to be attempted?

Anxiety is a bigger threat to my wellbeing than thrombocytopenia.
Is healing a matter of patience?
Is it about letting myself have bad days?
Is it, rather, knowing that a day is never bad in itself,
and I need only be gentle with my expectations?
How can I possibly heal without medicine?
How can we have let that word, medicine,
take on so narrow an understanding?
What happens when the pharmacy does far more harm than is its due?
Are there ways to heal that come with no pain, no suffering?
Is there such a thing as medicine without side-effects?

It's as if birth itself is the fall, towards death, the horror.
Rather my body is always in the process of composing itself.
As the cosmos is alive and populated by mystery,
I live into the creation myth while my body cycles back around
sickness, healing, growth, decay.

The documents in my archive of care create a linear fiction of treatment.
A correspondence of actors playing out their role in the narrative:

The fall, in which sickness occurs.
   Diagnosis, treatment, so much drama.
And the resolution around which the narrative is formed:
   recovery.
After which I ought to thank my tireless experts,
because a teen spokesperson for the appropriate
   Rare Illness Support Association,
and run a marathon fundraiser in order to prove
   that I overcame,
got my Normal Body back, and with enough determination,
   you too can Recover.
Of course some, perhaps many, sick people, want to not be sick any more.

But this seems like a misunderstanding.
We do not desire a return to normal,
We only want joyous embodiment.
Never in their lives would the doctors venture
autoimmunity as a positive experience.
Always, it is merely another reason to manage the occulted body.
Chemical technologies of control to regulate
an autoimmune system which
in my apprehension of life
exceeds the merely material.

Cure is a myth, where returning to "before" collapses
the imperative linear time and reveals inner cyclicality.
Auto-immunity shatters the telos upon shores of blood.
It is time itself, not our bodies, that is sick.
It is the clock as master and metaphor,
that British imperial naval technology,
which wreaks havoc upon our flesh.
It is not cure you want. It is rest.
What your body desires is an exit from alarm clocks,
and a rhythm of its own. Our cells breathe at their own pace.
It's a withdrawal from the incessant poison of empire that heals.

I suppose I am in search of a cure. That's the 'reward' around which I've been orienting my life, my striving. Unconsciously. Would it be better to seek cure consciously? Or to strive for acceptance and reconciliation with what is?

I love this flesh; it is all I know. Sorry: that it must harm itself. Grieving for the blood shed inward. For why must a body be toxic? In that question the endeavour: How is the human body made toxic?

A record of treatment turns the ongoing chronicity of healing into a past cure, a fait accompli. The slew of blood tests fixes a fictionally static count of my body in time where a living organism is always shifting and responding to worldly cycles

I have not spontaneously ceased this mode of self-defence. I have not entered a new realm of embodiment by changing locales and breathing new air. My existence is essentially continuous. I may not know where I'll end up, or even where I'm going, but for the time being I sense that I'm doing what I can to live a life of truth, harmony. Not pushing needlessly in a direction that won't have me, but feeling in the dark for those secure handholds, where a latch awaits my touch. I do not mean that the path must be easy--rather, that it must carry that distinct feeling-tone of rightness.

All I really know is that I wake up each day, thankful for the gift that is life. I am assailed by doubt and uncertainties. What is there to ensure that the world has meaning? I choose to believe the order has its own reason, which I may never grasp. The human answers do not satisfy me, even when those lives ordered by such stories appeal greatly.. The only certainty is the is-ness of flesh. Through this is, the world is sensed in turn. Sensation is divine nature, the great teacher. Confusion is an aspect of the flesh, when the grandeur of sensing relations overwhelms the conscious. The flesh itself knows no limits, and may perceive the oneness of is-ness when left to sense without interference from my mind.

This is why it pains me to ingest pharmacology's product. It stretches and expands the flesh according to logics I do not comprehend. It activates my body as if it were separate from the mind--leaving me to make sense of the flesh's entangled nature all on my own. I am furious at the lack of guidance afforded me. None explain their reasoning: Recommendations come as blanket prescriptions, as band-aids. Is no one looking causation, for cure? Am I?

Reading Phaedrus
2021-02-26

Reading Plato because Simone Weil said he's a mystic.
Burnt through this quirky dialog.
Socrates and Phèdre lounge beneath an old tree
to ponder Love+Language.

What is the role of madness in love?
They find that amorous impulse is driven by Aphrodite and Eros,
and this divine compulsion is the greatest form of madness.

This, as counterpoint to the opening
with Lysias' take against the man-in-love,
cast as one who must not be trusted
for he can not act in mutual best-interest
when under the influence of love.

I'm pleasantly surprised by the ever-presence of gods
as well as the relationship dynamics of greek men
who clearly understand that ecstasy is to be found in the flesh.

Is followed by a less interesting section
on the foundation of rhetoric and dialectical method.

1- Pick a subject
2- break it down into composite parts
3- Define those elements in such a way as to advance your argument.

Is that what I'm doing here?

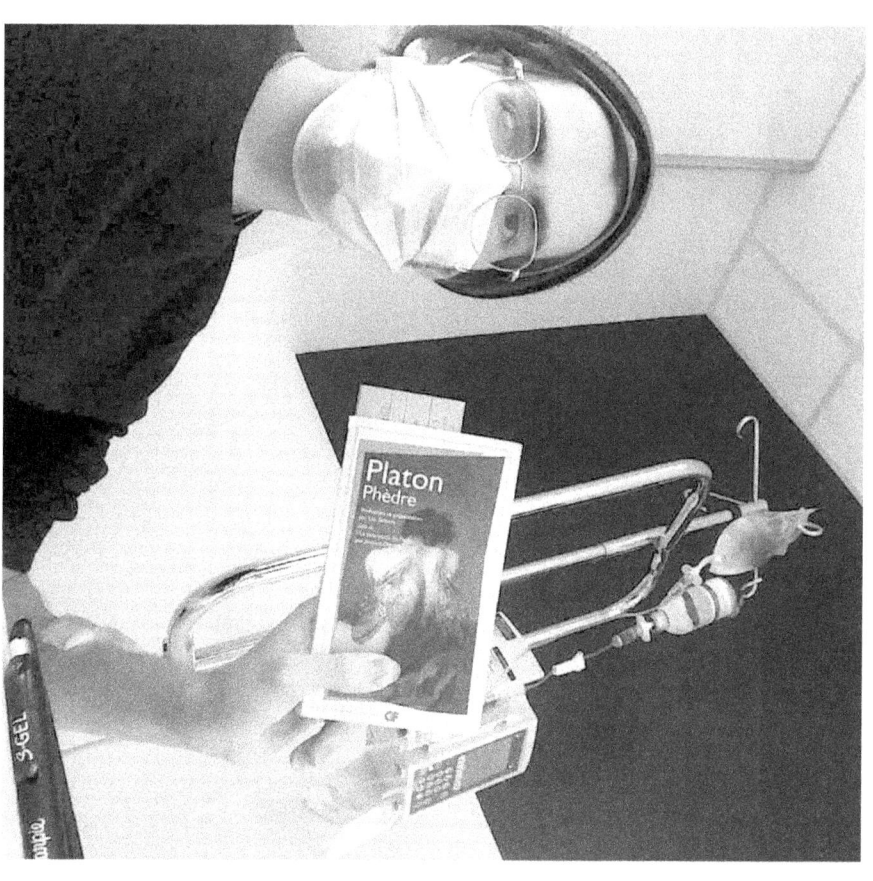

Vein To Vial

THE TOPIC HERE IS a common medical intervention

Human blood plasma gets extracted,
    processed into a commodity,
and administered through intravenous transfusion.
Plasma becomes Privigen®,
and is used to treat the writer's thrombocytopenia,
so-called platelet deficiency.

Pathology: a risk for spontaneous internal bleeding.
Our plasma is part of my flesh, your flesh,
a liquid substrate of global haematology
the earth's collective lifeblood, the global bloodstream.

Thinking blood across individual realities,
draw out blood's complexity:
enfold family, state violence, and environmental racism
    into a gooey assemblage.
Science's narrow apprehension of materialist naturalism becomes
an embodied entanglement of history and experience.

My blood is more than just my own,
it is a collaboration, transits terrestrial arteries,
its nature shifts as it is harvested and becomes
    raw biological resource.
The blood-products resulting from extraction are charged
with the intergenerational relationships and trauma
having shaped the lives of people from whose bodies
    plasma is needled.

Privigen® is one blood product
   amongst a class of drug known as IVIG.
This particular "Intravenous Immunoglobulin (Human) 10% Solution for Infusion"
is manufactured by the self-styled
   Global Rare Disease Biotech Company, CSL Behring.
They harvest plasma in over 170 centres in the USA.

Consider that blood-derived-medicine exists through the mutually composed actions of so many people, places, ancestors, sciences, arts, histories, all acting within oneanother. Entanglements remain most noticeable at sites of transfer, where we open new territories. In situ: the bodies of plasma donors and plasma recipients.

The corporate elevator pitch:
Plasma is a Potent Weapon Against Diseases,
   A Life-Saving Solution,
which is Tracked Every Step Of The Way
Funnelled overland from Plasma Collection Centres
   across The Nation,
interstates flowing with cold-trucks keeping
   Plasma Testing Laboratories
and Plasma Logistics Centres
   in Knoxville, Indiana, and Mesquite, Texas,
supplied with the raw biological material
necessary for the occult practice of high-pharmacy.

> These logistics centres are state-of-the-art facilities for receiving, storing, and shipping plasma that is donated at our collection centres. The inventory is controlled by sophisticated software that is tied into our donor management computer system. The laboratories test millions of plasma samples each year, ensuring the safety of the plasma. We have vein to vial control, tracing each plasma unit from the initial donation, to laboratory test results, to logistics and on to the fractionation facilities—and ultimately the product made from the plasma you donate.
>
>   From CSL Behring's website

CSL's plasma donors are lured into donation
with a transparent value proposition:
Make Cash, Save Lives.

Inciting donations encourages people to willfully dispossess
   themselves of their plasma.
Interiority is drawn out and stretched
   across the global complexes of capital accumulation,
ongoing systemic oppression,
   and further encroachment, preying
upon the bodies most violated over the past millennium.
The plantation economy is reproduced,
and the poorest bodies are still harvested directly.

Pennies on the dollar are paid daily to thousands
across the USA lining up to "donate" their plasma,
in a mercantile bastardization of the gift.
One regular donor's blog post makes it plain:

> There's only one pro to donating plasma: the payment. The amount that you earn for donation depends on the current needs of the donor pool, but the highest paying plasma companies pay anywhere from 20-50$ per donation, and you can give twice a week!

Plasma extraction firms solicit a service from individuals
in the form of hours spent passively giving up
their body's naturally occurring vitality,
turns around to offer a product
   when it sells its drugs and blood.
Plasma centres are some of capitalism's
   most insidious mechanisms given form.
No longer does the system content itself
   with the exploitation of wage-labourers
who work to produce an inert product
   inherently alien to themselves.

A donor today is paid
roughly the same dollar amount for their plasma
as they would have been for their blood 90 years ago.
Donating plasma takes 2-3 hours per session.
So it transmutes to an hourly wage between 10-25$/hr.

> "The sellers of blood during the Great Financial Crisis who could not afford breakfast had to ward off fainting episodes once their bodies were down a pint. They knew well that cash gained through the commodification of blood can represent a loss for the body. From the outset, there were both volunteer and paid blood donors. [...] In New York, family and friends of patients were encouraged to donate, and individuals could earn $35 to $50 per donation. Given average annual income of around $1,200, the New York Times (February 11, 1923) labeled donating blood the "1,001st Way to Make a Living;" the donation price attracted people whose benefit from donating, from altruism and compensation, exceeded their costs (time, discomfort, and health risks)" (Slonim et al.)

   Just another gig.

Blood plasma is extracted from whole blood during donation
via a process called plasmapheresis,
which removes plasma and returns the remaining
red blood cells and platelets to the donor.

Since the 1960s,
   this process has decreased the health risks for donors,
making it possible to donate plasma as often as twice a week.
Whole blood is collected on a volunteer basis
   nearly worldwide
thanks to a variety of public initiatives.
Plasma, on the other hand, is in short supply.

At the turn of the 21st century,
   nearly 70% of the world's plasma
   originated from the United States.
It is also the only nation in the world
   to be self-reliant in blood and plasma products
thanks to a for-profit industry
that has evolved over a century.

In 2017, ABC Local News reported that

> the payment [donors] receive averages about $30 to $40, and for the companies, it is a $19.7 billion global industry.

Worldwide, public funds funnelled into healthcare systems
flow upwards to the multinational corporations
manufacturing the drugs used to treat the population:

> "Even with a largely voluntary supply of blood [...] hospitals pay for blood products and charge patients for their use. For example, the cost of the components of each unit of blood sold to hospitals in the United States is approximately $570, with the cost for red blood cells at $229, platelets at $300, and plasma at $40. Hospitals transfuse this blood at estimated costs of between $522 and $1,183 per unit in the United States and Europe." (The Market For Blood)

Gather up the canals of haematology's globalism
feel the heartbeat of the industrial machine
facilitating the care of patients
whose sick bodies need help.

Plasma collection is one profit-driven artery
rendering a pulse into a wholesale product,
constructing a multibillion dollar industry out of donations.
"Donors" appear as an undifferentiated class of people,
without accounting for the uneven distribution of risk
inherent to life within a decomposing leviathan.

Donors are all subject to pharmacopornographic apparatus,
wherein power's tendrils exist in the human body
through soft, bio-molecular technologies.

Healthcare is the pretense.
Health is the fiction mobilized each day.
Each of these is a moving part in my transcorporeality.

Time crawls as patients and donors cycle through my thoughts,
examine the clocks, distractions, infusion pumps
that tick tack whirr
and beep to mark different passings,
    asynchronous beats of the hum drum
clinical purgatory, impermanence sits
with the sense of imbibing
fluid hung from stainless steel,
served in pristine glass bottles
gently deflating sterile plastic sacs;
    the pump regulates flow,
making sure veins don't feast too fast.
Translucent saline solution opacifies the superstructures
inherent to contemporary cure, so observe the drip, drip,
drip, and forget that through the eye of the needle,
all this watery lifeblood was once yours,
is now mine, has always been ours.

The Sozialistisches Patientenkollektiv
    of the University of Heidelberg
turns illness into a weapon through their direct action.
Part of the 20th century's anti-psychiatry vanguard,
    they position
diagnosis as alienation
    and illness as the prerequisite and result
    of economic production.

Their tract for agitation reminds me that
    illness is the only available
    way of life under capitalism,
because medicine does not heal,
it merely provides an illusion of cure.
The hospital seeks the work-force rehabilitation
of ailing bodies
through systems for the management of health.

As it is, curing can never mean abolishing illness,
it means only restoring the patient's ability to work
    while we remain ill.

There exists a vicious cycle of Cured and Healthy.
Cured of illness, healthy again.
Healthy, but eventually in need of cure again.
Both are points of illness in time.
The practice of curing is focused on economic accumulation.
Healthy individuals are the byproduct,
capable of working until they need another cure
or they retire,
at which point they are likely to need cures more often,
to recover from the hardships of their career.

At 92 years of age, my grandmother explains to me:
"I've undergone more tests this year
than in my entire life prior.
As if we didn't know what the problem was.
They aren't testing for my wellbeing,
they're testing to create data."

Upon arrival on the website of Scantibodies Biologics,
one of many plasma extraction firms,
the visitor is offered the opportunity to
earn hundreds of dollars in exchange for
   a few hours a month spent donating.
Located in Southern California, Scantibodies
even offers bus rides to its centres
from the Mexican border, framing the service
as a casual/normal part of a day-trip
into the USA. Their FAQ emphatically sates:
YES! We offer FREE transportation to and from the San Ysidro border
   crossing for anyone who is wanting to become a donor or is already a donor.

On their homepage, I'm shown a white couple
   holding up reams of $100 bills
   with wide grins across their faces.
The choice of stock imagery serves
to hide the reality of the average person donating plasma:
primarily poor, working-class people of colour.
The precarious position of individuals
going to Scantibodies is showcased
by a local ABC News report,
whose journalist follows two black men with full-time jobs.
One man donates plasma in order to afford
a birthday gift for his daughter.
Another is unhoused,
living between shelters and a storage unit.

Scantibodies recruits its donors with advertisements
highlighting the ease and comfort
of the experience of donating.
Their message is *"Relax and enjoy our free WiFi!"*

Browsing the internet is as much a mechanism for
participating in the 24/7 attention economy
as it is a way of ignoring the reality of one's embodiment.

When I engage with online media platforms,
my taps and swipes and clicks generate revenue
for corporations and advertisers.
Jonathan Crary remarks that

> The more one identifies with the insubstantial electronic surrogates for the physical self, the more one seems to conjure an exemption from the biocide underway everywhere on the planet. At the same time, one becomes chillingly oblivious to the fragility and transience of actual living things.
>
> 24/7

Scantibodies assumes, knows,
that people enjoy the internet enough
to forget or ignore that their lifeblood
is being extracted for profit.
Relax, enjoy the wifi, have a juice,
this will only take an hour or two,
you can leave cash-in-hand, go shopping,
and get a complementary bus ride back home.
What a deal.

Moving from vein to vial,
plasma is only accessible when
carefully drawn from human bodies
by trained professionals
using industrial medical equipment.

There is no synthetic plasma manufacturing process
to replace the human body as a source of raw material.

Plasma on its own is a straw-colored liquid that carries
red blood cells, white blood cells, and platelets.
It's made up of water (90%),
proteins and clotting factors (8%),
and small amounts of salts, sugars, and fats.

The building blocks of flesh are those nutrients
found in food, air, water, dirt.
Bloodlines mingle with the chemico-industrial assembly-line,
and the results of plasma harvest are
    condensed into Privigen®,
to be slowly assimilated by vampiric bodies down the line.

Intravenous Immunoglobulin products are prepared
from the serum of between 1000 and 15000 donors per batch.
Privigen®'s product monograph states that it is
"prepared from large pools of human plasma."

Donors and patients are brought together
by the mobilization of liquid resources originating
not in "nature" but alchemized by the human body itself.

Donors are unknowable and numerous.
IVIG exists through passages among bodies,
single-use needles, tubes, plasmapheresis machines,
laboratories, de-pathologizing agents, sterile bottles,
warehouses, cross-border transport, hospitals and clinics
worldwide. Plasma continually takes on a new liquid form
dictated by its position and its vessel, sloshing about
and freezing solid, always carrying its multiple biographies.

By the time IVIG reaches the clinic
and hangs above an infusion pump,
plasma is part of a "clear or slightly opalescent,
colorless to pale yellow solution,
a highly purified product."
The processes involved in the manufacture of Privigen®
are a series of attempts on the part of medical science
to strip plasma of its specificity
as part of an individual human's bloodstream.
An attempt to create a thing from a person.
Materialist reductionism at its finest cutting edge,
the creation of a distinct resource subject to human control.

The assembled liquid becomes Privigen®
by a trick of the word,
an immaterial coercion imposed upon molecular soup.
In naming Privigen® as Privigen®,
word and flesh are inextricable.
An incorporeal change which creates medicine,
while plasma harvest makes Privigen®'s "human"
a misnomer, a trick. Plasma is extracted from human bodies,
but exists only through scientific apparatus.

The language of Privigen®'s monograph is couched
in a tacit erasure of histories shaping who gets to be
Human, what gets to be A Person.
The blood-product does not shed these histories
as it it undergoes biochemical treatment and traverses
international and transcorporeal borderlands.
Taken together, this veinous pathway of the global bloodstream
makes possible the care of patients.

Patient bodies are made docile through soft coercion;
frictionless adoption of medical treatment is demanded
habitual acceptance of medical authority develops over time.

To the best of its bureaucratic ability,
a hospital hierarchically decides which bodies are prioritized.
Enacting carceral affinity for continuous inspection,
hospitals have come to be defined by their precise investigation
of bodies and deployment of strategies to manage them.
Hospitals ensure the careful tracking of a body's state,
and construct bodies as bureaucratic data
through their management processes.
Each change in a patient's bodily state is recorded
in order to trace their progress and determine suitable ministrations.
Stressors are kept to a minimum,
patients are sheltered with great care.
In exchange for the privilege of accessing the hospital space
within this tax-payer funded healthcare system,
patients are asked only to abide by certain regulations.
In return for services rendered the task of the patient is, simply, to get better.

While donors and patients were previously cut off
from the noise for the duration of their duties,
internet access provides them with continued involvement
in their personal reality-portal to the outside, always accessible.
The advent of wifi is potentially liberating to patients,
whose media diet is opened up to endless choices (in theory).

In the last decade,
and particularly with the advent of modern super-hospitals
such as Montreal's new multibillion dollar
Centre Hospitalier Universitaire de Montréal,
WiFi has become available to patients,
allowing freedom of media consumption
unlike any time prior
(for certain segments of the patient population.)

When hospital rooms were solely equipped with televisions,
many hospitals charged a fee for access
and controlled TV usage on a per-patient basis.
This practice allowed people of a certain means
to keep up with the goings-on of the outside world,
while those unable to pay the fee
(or for whom the fee was not covered under health insurance)
were relegated to cold media, slow media.

Obsession with data follows a long tradition
of building disciplinary practices into therapeutic spaces.
The tracking of patients, the act of
turning their bodies into data,
has been at the foundation of healthcare
since the first modern hospital opened
in the 18th century.

Next time you're at a hospital, pull out your smartphone.
Try to get off on the public wifi. Report back.
Did it work?

I checked and can confirm that all websites
labeled 'Pornography'
are blocked on the hospital WiFi in Montreal's Nouveau CHUM,
that glass skyscraper complex by Champ-de-Mars metro.
Who decided inpatients shouldn't be allowed to watch smut?
Inpatients specifically, because anyone else passing through
has the option of accessing internet elsewhere,
after their clinical visit is over. The hospital is ever a disciplinary space.
There are ways in which patients get around the barriers
baked into the public WiFi network. For anyone raised online,
or anyone with a data plan
it's easy enough to subvert the SysAdmins,
find websites that elude detection.

A doctor in my extended family says that the rules are in place
to restrict misbehaviour by staff, the doctors themselves.
Apparently it's all too common for them to fuck each other
between patient visits, in the examination rooms.
Is anyone surprised? But how many inpatients know this?

The availability of Wifi may push the information gap further,
since a patient who is able to use a device with internet access
can lead a 'normal' existence,
and one without access to or skill with the technology is
effectively disabled by the infrastructure,
and must rely on word of mouth for news and information
about the outside world.

The literature I was able to find about wifi in hospitals
focused on the ways in which the technology could be used
to track the movements of patients within the institutions,
I guess contact tracing was nothing new.

In my conversations about hospitalization,
friends seem endlessly surprised to discover
that people are widely left to their own devices
during their time as patients, yet media consumption
has been a central part of hospitalization
for as long as I have been a patient.

Most hospital rooms were equipped with televisions
for easy distraction,
but ultimately my choice of activity
depended on my energy levels.
Certain tasks simply require more stamina than others.

Being a patient is work
it interferes with expectations of productive labour.
Despite this, sick people still need to "earn a living,"
and continue to engage in the labour, paid and unpaid,
of the late-capitalist 24/7 economy.

A patient with internet access can socialize,
work, and engage with the world's happenings in realtime
"Since no moment, place, or situation now exists
in which one can not shop, consume, or exploit
networked resources, there is a relentless incursion
of the non-time of 24/7 into every aspect
of social or personal life." (Crary again)

The existing literature treating internet usage by hospital inpatients
deals primarily with increasing patient engagement
of online health portals.
In 2015, a survey examined the use of mobile devices
among hospitalized patients in a large urban Californian hospital,
with the goal of determining how many patients

a) brought devices to the hospital with them, and
b) used their devices to access their personal health record.

This paper says that 68% of surveyed patients brought
at least 1 mobile computing device,
the largest determining factor for device use was age,
rather than insurance status or race/ethnicity.

79% of people under the age of 65 used a device,
27% of people over 65 did.

48% of device users accessed their health data,
79% of device users used their device for 'entertainment/games'

The authors do not expand on what is meant by 'entertainment/games'
As of writing, no further surveys have been conducted
which examine the ways in which hospitalized patients spend their time online.

In practice, the advent of wireless internet in hospitals is a relinquishing of control
over the channels of information available to patients.
Caregivers no longer need to manage media consumption on top of healthcare.
The internet acts as a pacifier, a thumb stuck in the mouth,
providing distraction from embodied experience
and facilitating willful amnesia about pain and sickness,
which lessens the burden of emotional labour the nurses must exert.

In Surveiller et Punir, Michel Foucault made explicit the "force secrète"
which alleges a mandate of personal betterment for its subjects.
   Meaning: Discipline Helps You Get Better
The exertion of biopower is nowhere more visible than in hospitals,
which create an isolating environment
allegedly suitable for bodily healing,
rather than isolation in the name of punishment.

> "L'isolement constitue un 'choc terrible' à partir duquel le condamné, échappant aux mauvaises influences, peut faire un retour sur soi et redécouvrir au fond de sa conscience la voix du bien"
>
> Surveiller et punir, p.145

Are the sick condemned to repent?
The insular nature of the hospice bed
cuts off the inpatient from the outside
and its 'unhealthy' atmosphere.

It is in the name of cure, the betterment of patients,
that a sick body is processed and tracked.
A body must be on its best behaviour
in order to undertake the necessary labour of rest and repair.
Hospital time is unfixed—shifting dependent on a body's receptivity to cure.

With regard to internet usage,
the policies are framed as being in the best interest of patient health,
yet make an implicit moral judgement about pornography
and about the sexuality of patients.
It seems to me that the restriction of pornography
amounts to an important barrier of the potential
for a sexual identity among hospitalized patients.
The browsing restrictions built into the public WiFi
serve as a moralizing proscription on the rights of adults
to access legal materials online,
as well as a prohibition of their identities as sexual beings.

The restrictions surrounding pornography in the hospital
serve to further stigmatize groups of people already touted as asexual,
and prevent patients from a common avenue
for sexuality, should they desire to engage.

The hospital's mission is explicitly
to promote health and well-being.
They aim to "facilitate healthy choices",
"lead meaningful interventions",
and facilitate "free and enlightened decision-making."

That means condemning behaviours and habits
that may be detrimental to mental and physical wellness.
The public conversation's effacement of sexual pleasure
as a valuable part of daily life works hand-in-hand
with the dominant view that chronically ill people
could not possibly be concerned with sexuality
to create a habitat that doesn't think twice about denying
its residents access to sexually explicit materials.

Bodies learn behaviours and habits when led by example.
Here, bodily discipline is enforced by creating barriers to sexually explicit material
obviously linked with masturbation and sexual pleasure.

There are reams of papers showing that in clinical contexts,
pornography consumption is restricted to sanctioned medical uses
such as research or "sexual rehabilitation" programs.

Power over the acts permitted an individual is central
to the formation of docile bodies;
disciplinary power creates a correlation
between action and state of embodiment:
"le contrôle disciplinaire ne consiste pas simplement à enseigner
ou à imposer une série de gestes définis;
il impose la relation la meilleure
entre un geste et l'attitude globale du corps" (p.178)

Discipline of embodied gestures is inextricably linked
with the betterment of a body's behaviour.
In the case of health, if pornography is unhealthy,
then one must not be allowed to consume this poison
when attempting to cast off other ills,
or healing as a whole is jeopardized.

> "La punition est une technique de coercition des individus; elle met en oeuvre des procédés de dressage du corps avec les traces qu'il laisse, sous formes d'habitudes, dans le comportement; et elle suppose la mise en place d'un pouvoir spécifique de gestion de la peine. Le souverain et sa force, le corps social, l'appareil administratif. La marque, le signe, la trace…"
> Surveiller et Punir, p.155

The patient's experience is also one of attempting
to forget one's position,
in order to allow time to pass more quickly.
One finds ways to distract oneself.
In my experience, every patient has their media of choice.
Reading, music, movies, games, social networks, work.
Anything goes.

Regular transfusion treatments and their side-effects
make it more difficult to reliably commit the time
that is demanded of the worker.
Hospitalization may force people to take
significant amounts of time off work,
if they are able to hold down a regular job.

IVIG further impinges on a patient's extra time,
compressing their opportunities for rest
into greater scarcity. The time carefully set aside
from work becomes time to catch up
on the productive obligations
that medical commitments trespass upon.
Being a patient is unpaid work;
work that often requires paying to access;
work that actively takes away the resources
acquired through productive labour.

Patients are expected to work on their health.
Crary's book frames its discussion around sleep,
which "in its profound uselessness and intrinsic passivity,
with the incalculable losses it causes in production time,
circulation, and consumption [...] will always collide
with the demands of a 24/7 universe."

Prior to internet connectivity, hospitalized time
functioned similarly to sleep vis-a-vis capitalism.

In the context of transfusions,
it is required that the patient remain passively
in place for the duration of the treatment
and allow their body to do the slow work of chemical absorption.

However, unlike sleep, the waking mind is still active during this time.
The patient is still a consumer, and with the arrival of WiFi
in many hospitals and clinics it has become possible,
perhaps necessary, for many chronically ill individuals
to perform two occupations simultaneously: patient and worker.

24/7 demands I forget about myself,
focus instead on the always-on world
of production and consumption.

The parallel procedures of donation and transfusion
are thus drawn together through internet access.
While the donors and patients are alienated from their bodies
by necessity, either for money or for cure,
they engage in the legible act of consumption.

If there's no getting better, patients learn to work through it.
For people who are at the hospital regularly,
it is not a vacation or an opportunity to focus on healing.
It is a part of the routine that must be accounted for
in one's crip-time management. One may ask oneself:
"how much time do I need off work each month for this,
for the foreseeable future?"

Alison Kafer meditates on 'prognosis time', calling it

> "a liminal temporality, a casting out of time; rather than a stable, steady progression through the stages of life, time is arrested, stopped. Paradoxically, even as the very notion of 'prognosis' sets up the future as known and knowable, futurity itself becomes tenuous, precarious. But this very precariousness can [...] become an impetus for erotic investment in the present, in one's diagnosed body."
>
> Feminist, Queer, Crip, p. 36

To invest oneself in the present, in embodied experience,
is a fundamental departure from capitalism.
Paying attention to the material realities of treatment
and the immediate situation, rather than ignoring them
and hoping they pass, is a radical form of acceptance.

In the hospital chair of a WiFi-enabled institution
the networks of crip time and 24/7 careen into one another
within one sick millennial's laptop open to messenger.

Waiting
2021-04-10

I'VE BEEN WAITING FOR waiting to happen.
And what do I do while I wait?
Get dragged into computing habits staring at a screen
watching television eyes burning into my sockets.
Smoking cannabis passing the time reminding myself
that waiting for the sake of waiting is not necessarily time lost.
Journaling and omitting to transcribe,
not really sure what to do now
that certain projects are in another's ballpark.

Hello, is anyone out there?
What do you think?
What do I think?

I think I have to keep practicing
and apply myself for the sake of myself,
not apply to work useless jobs.

Would be nice for my days to feel substantial
but I can settle for early mornings
out by the water moving what little qi I have.

Frustrated some days that I have no one to share with,
no teachers, no partners.
Only distant relations. No friends, really.

AUTO-IMMUNE HERESY

Sure, I know people, but what's a friend?
Someone with whom to build life and share knowledge.
The people now in my life are on paths
I find ultimately meaningless.
Is that cruel?

I suppose it's best that I find my own life
a more interesting affair than any other,
but that does not lessen the burden
of waking up and feeding myself, alone.

The weight of solitude turns me into a petty creature,
staving off boredom in what ways I can
I slowly develop an ascesis
that will lead somewhere worthwhile.

But in pandemic it feels like nothing is worth doing, somedays.
Even the most beautiful, the most powerful acts,
they fall short in my little solipsism.

Magic, meditation, breathing, movement,
the forest,
the water.
None of it helps.
Cannabis helps, but only for an hour or two.
That's not any good.
Mushrooms help, but imperceptibly.
Frustrating, frustrating.

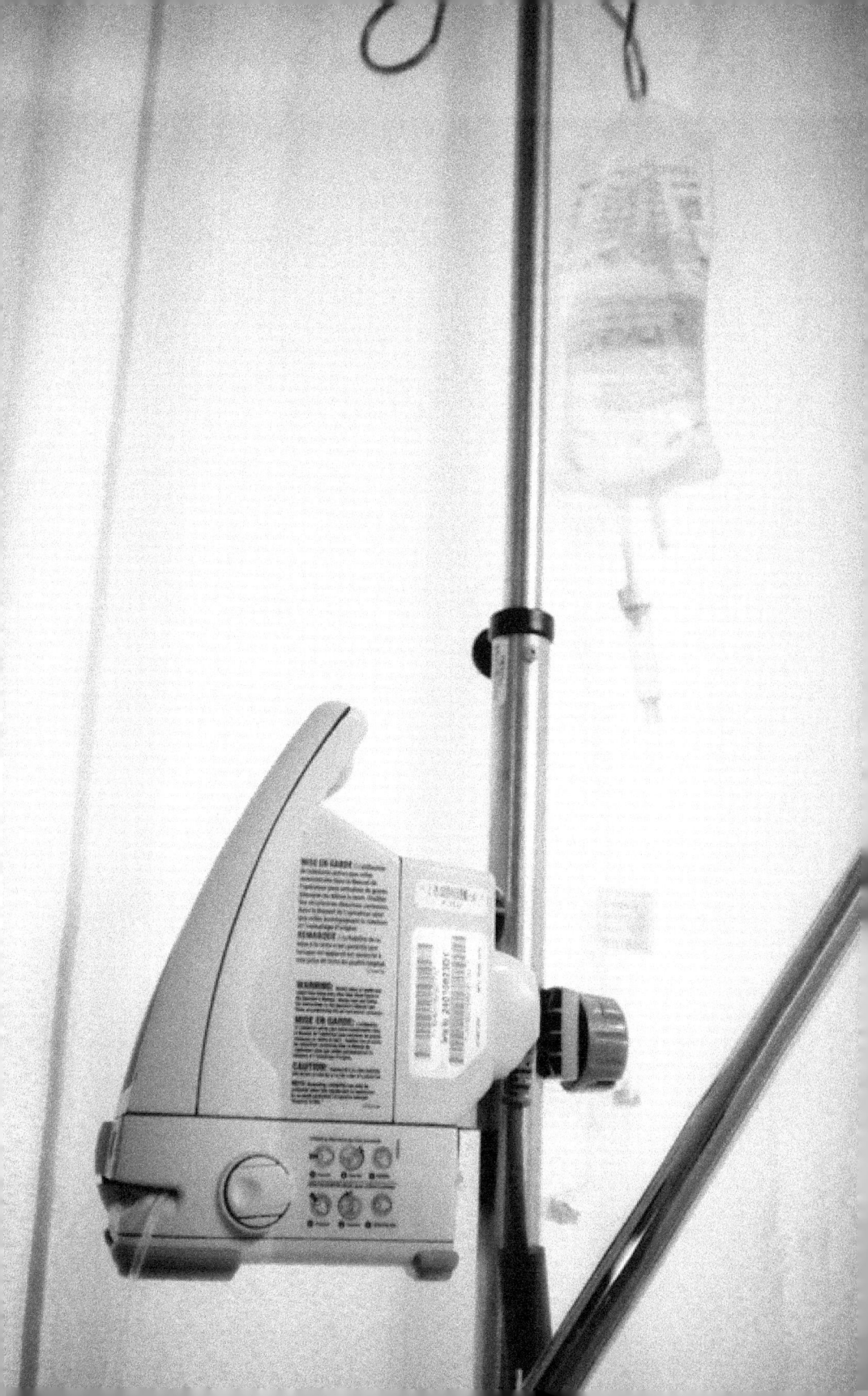

Vein To Vial, continued

But I digress, and
meanwhile, the needles do their own work.

Once the patient arrives for treatment,
a nurse measures body weight in order to determine
the speed and volume of the dose.
They prepare the intravenous catheter and ensure its proper functioning.
They program the pump, which is designed with the assumption
that its operators have a degree of medical knowledge
to allow them to make sense of its many features and safely operate it.
Nurses keep track of the infusion rate,
the liquid's volume, the patient's vitals.

Throughout the course of treatment, the pump and patient
are regularly monitored by a nurse. At specific intervals,
a patient's blood pressure and temperature are taken.
The process is not without risk, and common side-effects include
    dizziness, migraines, bodily pain, fever, and anxiety.

Due to the commonness of side-effects
during IVIG treatment, it is crucial that the patient
be carefully monitored for their own safety.
The nurse's role during the treatment is to
use their knowledge of medicine to actively track the data
generated by the pump and the patient,
as two machines to be monitored, checked on regularly—known to mal-
    function.

The nurse's view of the encounter is necessarily
colored by their medical training, years of practice
(or lack thereof),
and the relations of power that place
the nurse above the patient
in the hierarchy of knowledge,
but always below the specialist doctor
whose signature mandates the prescription.

Medical vernacular narrativizes illness as a fight,
as a war to be waged against and within one's own body.
I'll play along.

Expectations during transfusion echo those of combat.
While the patient is receiving IVIG,
invisible battles are waged at the cellular level,
their body is receiving a drop shipment of reinforcements.
Generals keep informed by monitoring data.
Meanwhile, the soldierly patient is caught in a skirmish
with the side-effects of their body's shifting
chemical (im)balance.
Vitals are assessed regularly by a nurse on duty,
monitoring the battleground.
The risks for the body are the driving factor
determining the rhythm of the encounter with IVIG.

Bloodiness is a magnetism, an earthiness.
Observing my own arms the veins are hills and tunnels.
They bulge and recess in turn.

It's commonplace for a nurse in a talkative mood
to comment upon their quality.
Expert appraisal has it: my veins are ripe for needling.
Not that any of us are too eager.
They're working, sticking needles into veins for days on end.
Sick work, bloody labour.
Most nurses are highly skilled at this task.
Commendable. It barely hurts.

The unpredictable nature of IVIG side-effects
demand an awareness of one's own existence in the world,
coexisting with the machines,
the drugs, and the nurses all around
and all implicated in the happening.
At a given moment during the transfusion,
the body might refuse the medication.
In spite of this, the patient is not expected
to take an active part in the process.
The body only receives.
Much as plasma donors are invited to 'relax with free wifi!',
the patient is asked to sit back, breathe,
and allow the requisite time to pass.

Back into human corporeality through a new needle,
down the intravenous drip from the infusion pump
and the sterile containers.
The crystalline substance comes into
another biological body at last.

Not for the first time, not for the last time,
I soak up it all up.

Frame a photograph, click, freezing the drip...drip...drip...
Sitting cannulated, plenty of places I'd rather be,
sat in a blue chair within blue walls
bleeding red in purple veins
while crystal clear plasma fractionations
make up the difference.

The human body and blood-product collide
in their inescapable urge to merge,
the global bloodstream's capillaries meeting in transfusion.

Fusion, underscoring the loss of discrete identities
between the concoction and the body,
implies oneness and indissolubility.

Privigen® soon disappears and turns "Human" again
within new veins. Co-mingling
with this new host, plasma-cum-Privigen®
finds a body different from the thousands it inhabited
in its past lives. Plugged into the infusion pump,
the patient submits their human body
to the clinical environment. The assimilation
is accompanied by an array of multisensory reactions.
The experience of transfusion confers
a uniquely embodied knowledge,
and the patient's body must successfully
assimilate, or reject the drug.

A needle is a tool,
manufactured to transit blood into the realm of medicine:
use, examination, engineering, processing, alteration.
In opening a vein, the needle has served
its utilitarian purpose.
As blood moves through the needle into a world of industry,
the needle comes into being through
a narrow technoscientific focus.
A transitory, ephemeral vessel for blood,
designed as a single-use object.
A sterile puncturing device made of steel,
wrapped in plastic,
only useful in conjunction with innumerable
operative relations
specific to the bloodstream's global assemblage.

As soon as blood has sufficiently flowed,
withdraw the needle and dispose of it.
Throw it away into that specially marked
fluorescent-yellow bin: biohazard.
So the needle's journey continues into trash-heaps
and landfills; tubes touched by human blood
are too dangerous for recycling.

Nothing opens or closes this bloodstream
the flow is uninterrupted, only the map changes.
Paths may shift but assemblages, in all their specificities,
enact the relations which create words and flesh,
dirt and water, none of which are discrete.
Blood is the substance of human life,
othered by its capture into the industry's web.

On this map, the intravenous needle is the site of othering.
In Deleuze and Guattari's terms,
it is the machine which holds the key,
the cutting edge inserting itself into the donor
(full of its all-too-fleshy organs, already organ-less,
blood-less, mere raw material for sale),
drawing out essence from a single organism
to a node within the planetary bloodstream.

In the acts of needling and blood-draw,
blood is uprooted from its origin within the donor's porous body
and seeps into the territories of biotechnology
and medical industry.
It becomes plasma.

Hydration and medication and nutrition share an entry point,
a singular superficial vein in the arm
or the wrist or the hand.

Privigen®'s product monograph states that
"the recommended initial infusion rate of Privigen® is
0.5 mg/kg/min. If well tolerated, the rate of administration
may gradually be increased up to an infusion rate of 12 mg/kg/min."
Let's pause for some quick math. I weigh approximately 60 kilograms.

60kg x 2g = 120g or 120'000mg.
Maximum rate of infusion: 12mg/kg/minute
12mg x 60kg = 720mg per minute
x 60 minutes = 43200mg per hour
120'000mg total divided by 43'200mg/hour = 2.77 hours
At the maximum rate of infusion, the treatment takes just under 3 hours.

Now the minimum: 0.5mg/kg/minute
0.5mg x 60kg = 30 mg per minute
x 60 minutes = 1800 mg per hour
120'000mg total divided by 1800mg/hour = 66.666... hours
Or, roughly 67 hours.

So, IVIG may take me between 3 and 67 hours to receive, per dose.
The reality is somewhere in between, since the rate fluctuates
In my experience, infusion took somewhere between 4-8 hours,
without taking into account the logistical considerations
of other appointments, tests, and the fact of getting to the hospital.

The bags of fluid hanging over the pump empty out
and get replaced many times daily.
Sometimes they are medicine, sometimes they are
simply to keep the cannula from clogging.
Passive, the body becomes a chemical battleground
for armies of vastly different scales while the
mind occupies itself with other tasks.
Unpredictable details of experience demand an awareness
of one's own existence in the world, collaborating with the machines,
the drugs, and the medical professionals all around
and all implicated in the global flow of blood-derived-medicine.

How do I live transfusion?
Each donor gives something essential with their plasma.
There is more than a material transfer of blood proteins happening.

24 HOURS AFTER TREATMENT, the migraine hit. Beneath the cacophony of pressure pulsing in my skull I hear words, fragments of thought, worries and concerns: suicide; hunger; poverty; last resorts. Transfusion sends me spiralling through the night sky above Nepal. Alive, dancing a transient prayer in trance before a kneeling idol. Venus burns above. Lust seethes and bares its teeth, leaving fire trails of crimson until control is relinquished willingly. Then each bite tears away a part for itself, hungry ravenous flesh but not yours alone. We need variety at this table if we are to dine joyfully. Dust flies with step of the dancer's bare feet. Communion intensifies and each participants feels the Arrival of death and love. Spiralling, to make known that this body belongs to them. Please, they ask, allow me to gouge out your eyes, to enact the lessons of pain. Gouging must occur without anaesthetic of amphetamines of the kinds you give your soldiers. I'll keep you isolated in a room with only the minimum necessary sustenance, have you reach the ground-state of sobriety. Don't worry, you'll survive. I haven't decided whether to use a fork or a spoon, which would you prefer? Open your eyes, the nurse tells me, the treatment is over for today. Tell me you miss me. Tell me how our distance is hurting you. Tell me how your skin longs for mine. Tell me how your eyes hunt for mine. Tell me I'm enough of a woman for you. Tell me my anger is okay. Tell me you understand. Tell me my fear you love me less is unfounded. Stop telling me about other people, you're the only one that matters. Tell me your heart hurts too. Show me, rip out your sternum and tear apart your thorax and show me. Burning in my chest, our distance subsides to hollowness when the fire dwindles. I wish I could scream and wail and break my mirror and immolate my bones if only to make the feeling dissipate if only to make you go away if only if only if only it could turn to warm sadness I try to follow to its source that turns to rage again. Frustration. Would that I could rip out my valvular pump and hold it up to my cornea, if looking is truly the most effective way to Know. Broad daylight, sun pierces through the canopy of broadleaf deciduous life. A harsh metal scrape and the tearing of wood. Push, pull, push, pull. A human-powered deforestation, saw in hand. Mechanically we chant to keep the cadence, but I do not hear my own voice. The tree interpellates me. What are we doing? Why take by metallic force instead of asking for help? Don't we know that our larghissimo elders, the birches, the cedars, the maples, are ready to fall on their own if we speak the right words? But I do not heed this train of thought. The saw shakes in my grip and the tree is finally felled. Would that I could freeze time and devote endless life to understanding pain's anatomy. This pain is not my longing for you, though my longing is there subsumed.

AUTO-IMMUNE HERESY

This pain is bigger than I am, and narrow as a platinum razor's edge. A pickaxe in hand. Heavy beneath an empty stomach I dig at the grave I will inhabit soon enough. I do not know when the end arrives. I ask myself whether my grandfather was right to fear death. At least I will get to stop digging. Nearby, a young man, younger than me, grey with fatigue, falls. I await the inevitable order: Oi! Heb das auf, stapel es mit den anderen. I do not complain, merely comply, do not meet the soldier's eyes. They lead nowhere I wish to go. Hier la transfusion m'emmena à Kathmandou, il y a 12 générations. L'ancêtre sanguin se fit connaître. Je danse en prière devant une croupissante idole. Vénus brûle au-dessus de moi, et je danse. Un cercle fiévreux se forme au rythme de mon corps. La poussière virevolte à chaque pas que prennent mes agiles pieds nus. La communion s'intensifie, et tous nous ressentons l'Arrivée d'une déesse de l'amour et de la mort. Je tourbillonne, je dois être à sa hauteur, lui faire savoir que mon corps est sien, qu'elle n'a qu'à me prendre dans ses bras. These words are neither me nor not me, not any more or less than the ten thousand souls that inhabit me. The words: the plasma of thousands within my veins. Unknowable, yet pained. It is a matter of soul. Too much, too many. Pressure builds. Only so much can be processed at once. Clogged up with so many essences. The first 16 hours are the most revelatory. I know during that period just how alive the plasma remains, dripping from the flask. My blood is aflame, I run a fever. The first time I stood up, I thought perhaps a lifetime had gone. Every step riddled with latency, raising a thermometer takes eons. My vision is blurry, noisy. Each twitch of a muscle clatters. Standing is akin to shattering a mountain. I find myself praying. First to Abraham's God. Then Michaël, Raphaël. Then my grandparents. Then I beseech those souls directly coursing in my veins. I address them, plead for respite. Despite being of the blood, they remember little of the pain of flesh. So it was that my body recognized them, and did all in its power to remember suffering on their behalf. The following night I dream long, beautiful dreams full of longing. For place, for company, for shared meals. We argue warmheartedly over what to get at the store. I float through the storeroom. It was dark except for the flood of street-lamps through makeshift curtains and we both scream ecstasy. Rolling over once the high leaves my muscles, touch reverts to terror. How many times did I push them away when I wished to hold us close? The weight of their body felt crushing upon arms chest gut—any pressure brought a flood of fear. What if arteries pop veins rip flow ceases? My lover's head resting upon my chest brings it all back, the irrational bleeding mind, assailed by bodily doubt, harrowing anxieties.

Memories of dark purple bulbs, protrusions and all any of us know of them is bleeding. On a long bus ride, a friendship is forged in philosophy, a bond of lovers. Ecstasy again awakens me and I find the migraine mostly gone. So IVIG induced an experience of the sublime. It might be an entheogen. One body is no proper container for thousands.

Hiromu Arakawa's Fullmetal Alchemist
is worth its weight in salt, sheer joy
at the honest love and hate of characters at grips with truth.
If anyone wants to understand the experience of IVIG
they should try to understand Ed and Alphonse's dad, Van Hohenheim.

The process of transfusion is one by which medicine
turns Privigen® "human" again and creates
a homunculus of my body.

Every single donor
is my ancestor,
is my body,
is me.

I've been discussing the experiences of
donating plasma and receiving transfusions.
While I am critical of the corporate practices
with which these are intertwined,
I am not here to disparage the act of donating blood or plasma.

I acknowledge that the scores of people who donate,
compensated or otherwise,
are giving a gift to large swaths of the population.
I am perhaps alive because of you.
Giving blood facilitates life-saving medicine
on a daily basis.
The individuals involved in the blood economy
are engaging in essential actions
for those of us whose bodies
require regular or emergency assistance.

The fault does not reside within donation or transfusion.
These are simply material realities of medical practice.
The problem lies outside the classical frame of healthcare,
where capital interests muddy the waters
and turn healing into exploitation.

My goal is to offer another narrative,
one that runs parallel to that offered
blood donors and the public,
and in so doing, to shift perspective away
from dominant discourses of Health.

The healthcare system has a dual purpose:
it aims to rehabilitate sick people
so that they can get back to work,
and to maintain a relationship with the
medico-technical and pharmaceutical industries.

In doing so, the healthcare system acts
as the distribution centre of the medical-industrial
complex, simultaneously extracting money
from individuals and governments
for the benefit of corporations,
all the while "curing" people of their ills
so that they may return to producing surplus value.

Plasma Collection Centres choose to call
the sale of raw bodily material a donation,
linking it to the gift relationship with which people
engage for no monetary compensation.
The rhetoric reveals the industry's desire
to appear as a benefactor,
as falling in line with the purported
moral values of Healthcare.

I suggest we call these places Extraction Centres,
to be honest about the dividends demanded
from processing raw material.
Yet the firms do not market themselves
as extracting surplus value
from the bodies of their "donors."

Let's reorient perception of these companies
as driven by profit,
thus opening them up to a certain critique.
By aligning themselves with Healthcare,
a plasma extraction firm renders its operating strategy opaque.
According to the rhetoric employed,
the system in place grants "donors" the privilege of doing good work.
Technoscientific capitalism would have its subjects believe that
it is not at fault for making it necessary that low-income individuals
supplement their bottom-line by selling plasma.
The onus of choice is apparently placed on the individuals "donating,"
but many living in precarity have no other remaining options
but to sell their own flesh.
The moral sledgehammer falls heavy.
Make cash, save lives.

American human-hours in the form of blood
trickle downwards through the global medical-industrial complex.
Opposite the upward flow of taxpayer dollars
in public healthcare systems buying plasma-derived drugs

In extracting plasma for profit, corporations are
continually alienating poor working class people from their own bodies.
On the receiving end, the opaque nature of medicine works to pacify
the patients whose lives depend on an indefinite supply of transfusions,
and what is taken from the ill person is
their urgent need to struggle for change.
In the end, patients rarely protest against
the destructive and exploitative nature of healthcare.
Donation and transfusion are counterparts,
concentrating human hours at opposite ends of the process,
operating in clinical environments on opposing subjects.

The seemingly solitary experience of transfusion
is an illusion
shattered by acknowledging that Privigen®
deposits thousands of unknowable donors within my bloodstream.

The extraction of plasma is already an act of alienation,
splitting apart the components of human blood
to harvest only that which is profitable.

The bodies at play are agents charged with their own histories,
but a patient is not necessarily aware of the systemic violence
and ongoing oppressions which create
the global bloodstream as an industry.

Patients whose wellbeing depends on
an indefinite supply of plasma
are often in the privileged position
of being able not to ask too many questions
about the functioning of the system
keeping their symptoms at bay.

The obfuscation of knowledge, the withholding,
may be crucial
to the operation of the healthcare industry.

If all the histories that charge Privigen® were known,
people might refuse treatment, hurt profits.

The dilemma runs deep: what's more important,
my own health, or that of 15000 impoverished "donors"?

That knowledge may also be too much,
for how can one body bear the violence
enacted upon thousands?

By taking an interest in transfusion,
and acknowledging the relationships
that are formed during the process,
a body regains agency,
and becomes a source of gnosis.

I was taught that my biology is not to be trusted.
The chemical decisions enacted in my
bloodstream were the enemy.

The language used by doctors to describe auto-immunity
makes it seem like there a civil war raging,
and the combatants are confused, engaging friendly-fire.

But that's not what's going on.
Auto-immunity is a recalibration, a warning.
A call to change habits, to listen closely to the invisible.
Healing does not come from microscopes and pharmacology.
The way out of autoimmunity is the composition of a new body.

Is there any truth to the proposition
that all our cells change every 7 years?

My body is a set of relationships
between the visible and the invisible.

A concerted effort has been sustained to render
ever more of it visible through imaging technologies.

But what about the other senses?
What about the corpuscles dedicated to sensing
chemical balance in the bloodstream?
What if those could be brought to individual awareness?
I say they can.

My cure is not medicine, it is knowledge becoming love.
Knowledge of my archive, of cell biology, of spiritual science, of quantum physics, of imperial histories, of medical politics, of settler-colonial genealogies, magic, and my own soul.
Integrated experiences of medical trauma,
loving kindness,
disillusionment.

A will to trust in my own body's capacity to heal
to move into another version of self,
one in which the pharmacy does not
dictate my realm of possibilities.

A will to devote myself to myself each and every day,
to learn how enmeshed my chemistry is with yours,

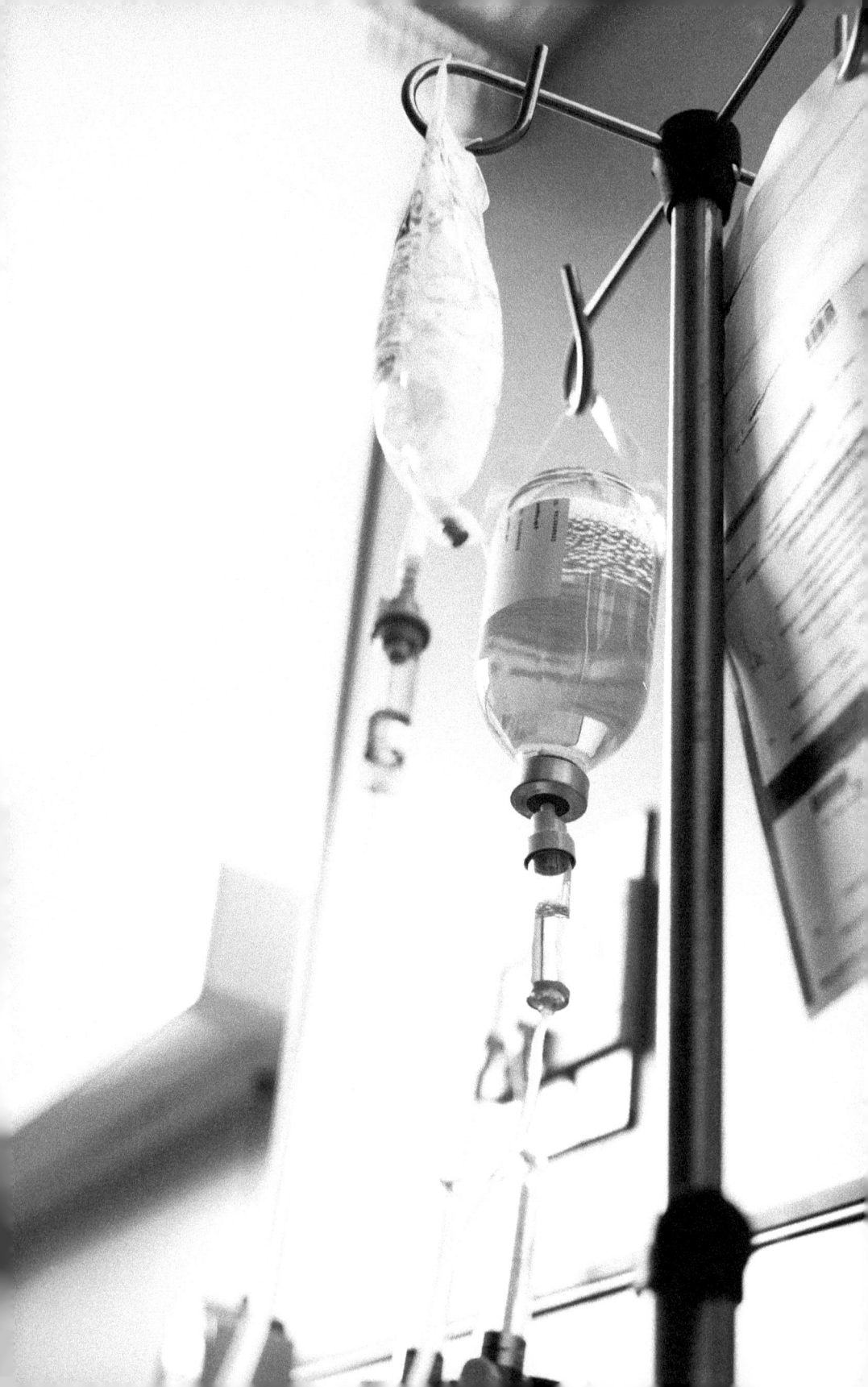

Sickness in Limbo

THROUGH THE NASCENT STORM, walk away from the river.
It's my first winter near my grandfather's grave,
on occupied territory first named Gespe'gewa'gi,
seventh district of Mi'gma'gi,
the ancestral and unceeded territory of the Mi'gmaq,
later christened Sainte-Anne-Des-Monts by my ancestors.
Seven-thousand inhabitants nestled
along the south bank of the St-Lawrence
49° North.
Here, on a clear day I can see the northern shoreline.
Here, I've learned that the wind is a fickle dance partner.
From the occulted beach, turn south.
Pace a side street amid bluster, foot after foot uphill in the snowdrifts,
towards the CLSC perched above town.
A reception clerk notifies the nurse of my arrival.
I sit in the waiting room.
I'm the only patient at first, but others soon arrive.

Today is March 5th, 2021, and I am still healing.
I await results, self-reparation.
What does the blood have to say, today?
I am repentant in the face of medicine,
I've come back after voluntary cessation of treatment.
I considered the immediate alternatives
and found the pharmakon I know will at least mitigate symptoms,
if never cure.

My intestines weep red and I wipe away tears alongside feces.
Now is not the time to gamble.
Patiently sit in a black plastic chair supported by a stainless-steel frame,
separate from the others visible through plexiglass bolted to the wall.
Postered on the wall there's a PSA about STI tests,
a showcase of lovers in ecstatic touch.
Matthieu-Xavier's name is called.
I pull my gaze away from the illustrated longing
and towards an old nurse named Thomas.
He's cheerful, deftly handles the needle.
His steady hands are the only human touch I feel each week.
We talk about the weather as he draws blood.
This winter, so he says, "has been exceptional, truly.
Exceptionally warm, and brief, and bereft of snow.
Trust me, this is nothing."

Before the time of remote friendships, in a limbo reserved for the sick,
I'm comforted by broken bread shared with others
    caught in their own ouroboros.
Each chronically healing body differs in its minutiae,
yet sickness breeds a hearth around which to gather and keep warm.
I reach out towards the fire, grateful for company that is not charity.
Grateful for those whose "I'm sorry" is not pity.
There is no pretence, no brave faces.
No imperative to cater to the comfort
of those who believe they are forever healthy.
I wager that for the sick, those who know that healing is cyclical,
a pandemic's disruption of time may have felt familiar.

This pandemic has shown me that
discussions of illness are no longer concerned with
the need to convince or remind the healthy that their certainty,
the self-assured confidence of perpetual health, is illusory.

The news media has done a thorough job of
instilling fear, breeding anxiety, and perpetuating
the poisonous narrative that is the hero's journey.

From healthy,
to sick, soon to be healthy again,
disease must be overcome.
Illness must be overcome.

So goes the story.
The calendar lies in tatters at my feet,
torn pages unstitched as despair and hope
enmesh in a spiral dance, a whirlwind
shreds my abdomen while delirium burns around me,
fear succeeds joy and, impatient to get a move on,
I dream of spring.

How long is a year, then?
Amidst a turmoil of organs, unsettled feuds remain.

Needled for a thousand blood draws,
I've come to reject the fiction of illness.

The global immune response to crisis
throws into sharp relief that healing is a learned skill.
There is no plotted course, no long-term plans,
but illness is not the only story,
and I devise strategies for a sick life.

I remind myself that healing goes on in illness,
that there is no miraculous cure-all.
Inner awareness, rest, and time off
are necessary tools for survival.

I am responsible for my own touch-starved self
and those few with whom I conspire.
I strive to tune into the resonance
by which I may make my way my own.

It begins when I listen to the flesh.
Then, breathe with the world and find myself
at home within the web of ongoing creation.
Stand still by the estuary
before the mouth of the river Sainte-Anne
as it pours into the St-Lawrence.
Ice shatters, sends waves up my spine,
and I know that the invisible flows
beneath the rustle of snow
are the same movements felt in my veins
and heard in the cracks of the ice.

Warmed by the sun under the vertiginous turquoise sky,
I give thanks for the chance to live such beauty
another day, another night.

COVID-19 will "end." The news cycles and feeds will move on.
What then? Will the transience of the body itself
have gained any respect?

Spring turns to summer
solar rays are talismanic but no protection
against the biting flies.
It is July 2021.
Deep in the forests of the Bas-Saint-Laurent,
stiff limbs shed fatigue as they awaken to use.
Months go by without a blood test.
Hands learn to craft metal and till the dirt.
I spend a week reworking a tin crucifix
into a solar necklace.
Rip Jesus off his cross.
Rend the soft metal into a new shape
and sand away decades of rust.
By the time I'm done it's a triangular pendant
with a soft gold sheen.
I give it to my grandmother,
the first piece of jewelry I ever made.

Black flies are unavoidable but plantain leaf
   makes an effective poultice.
I learn to walk, tread through the fields
   of foxtail and couch-grass,
     attuned to the pollinators whose hum guides my step.
Healing is of the dirt and water, my breath, my bones.
Healing is the love I hold for my body's proteins.
   Its ligatures, its fats, sugars, spinal liquidity,
     and all the microbes with whom I share these cells.
Healing is that peculiar sensation in the optic nerve
   confronted with sublimity,
     an old growth forest or an open sky.
The muscular jouissance of a footstep.
Sickness is in the chemical agonists at work on my spine's marrow.
Sickness is the rigidity of my fascia.
   I have so much to learn of healing from the trees,
   the birds, the frogs.
   The creak of limbs 50 feet above me,
   the withering bark, the barren branches.

Autumn, the black tar spot on fallen maple leaves,
the first scent of snow. The murder croaks at dawn.
The black birds are telling me to pray, to notice the decay.

Battered by winter, it is unclear
whether fatigue is physical or existential.
Or it is both.

I am an aquifer, from which Thomas' needle
   extracts groundwater.
Into the vial my blood flows,
examined for deficiency to track my risk of bleeding.
But sickness extends beyond the blood
it will not be contained by any such essentializing.
I am tackling the problem of healing in the long term.
Sickness, lived not as something to cure,
escape, climb out of, but as a maze
from which there is no exit, no future.

Healing is a labyrinth: it is the snake eating its tail.
Healing is acknowledging that Akeso
is too the daughter of Asclepius.

Treating such complexities with words,
in an attempt to cure pathology
according to numbers on a chart,
all this is too abstract.
Healing is anything but theory.
Without the imperative to strive
for a mythical life free from illness,
a sick existence breeds wondrous possibility.

I am armed with fresh clay through which I mold my body;
reams of blank paper upon which to compose symphonies.
The possibilities are not so remote. I choose to live
now the universal flourishing of an eternal recurring eden.
I am not in a circle of hell,
but a quiet place, a simple place.
Not the void, but somewhere to gather
and sing songs.

Thomas withdraws the needle,
affixes a small bandage to the leaky prick,
secures it with plastic medical tape.
I will wash off the gummy residue for three days.
I thank him and say, "see you next week."
Back outside, the blizzard has thickened.
Across the hospital parking lot,
I can't see the water in the distance.
I glean the outline of an oversized,
white-painted wooden cross planted at the cliff's edge.
On a clear day the visibility stretches for miles,
rounding the horizon.
So, I'm back to the walk, foot after foot,
down towards the river, north,
down the same path I followed up,
arm cradled to staunch the pinpoint wound,
curious whether today it will leave a bruise.

I do not refuse sickness,
I do not refuse the ongoing collapse
of so much I took for granted.
I strive for love in limbo and accept
that which I cannot control,
to better make meaning
from those minuscule decisions that shape each day.

I am doing things, moving by stillness.
I do all I can. The best with what is, right now.
The answers come only with time, unbidden, like old friends.
No right, no wrong. I am still healing.
I still take pills and attempt to make sense
of this body's enigma.
I know I am not alone in this, even if isolated in the cold.

A Spring Spent Nannying

I LEFT HOME TO the tune of Daydream Nation.
   She said: I wanted to map the exact dimensions of hell.
   Does this sound simple?

May 8th

"We're all gonna die! We're all gonna die!
Quick, take cover, get away from the acid rain."
In a military issue hammock nearby, khaki, green,
strung between a clothesline post and a young cedar,
I'm taking in the sunshine of high-spring
in the valley below Mont-Comi in the Bas-Saint-Laurent.
The horrendously joyous cackle nearby
the ode to impending doom
is the sound of children at play
on an oldschool trampoline, no safety netting.
They're huddled, yes,
under blankets, unzipped sleeping bags,
a fortress of their own design.
Limbs mustn't tresspass the protection of the game.
They all have enough to drink.
It arrives in the home via tap and consigned plastic jugs.
From the pipes, it sits in glass pitchers on the bar
to let some chlorine evaporate,
with no concern for heavy metals or pathogens.

Most mornings, they breakfast.
Eating any of the following, depending on their mood:
supermarket multigrain toast with butter,
white sugar cereal with milk,
cow's yogurt, fruit, or ramen noodles.
The eldest sometimes fasts, by choice.

May 14th

Dreamt of a matriarch's confession:
"I do not understand the world,
I made wrong decisions for posterity.
I have nothing for my kin."
The youth gather around her
petty, jealous, all thoughts on inheritance.

May 16th

Sat on a couch that each night serves as a bed,
eyes alternating between
Love In The Time Of Cholera
and the Gospel of Luke.
Thomas sits next to me, reading l'Agent Jean,
a Quebecois comic book for kids,
depicting the adventures of
a supergenius secret agent
anthropomorphic moose
named Jean, and
his wacky shenanigans
saving the world from absurd threats.
Thomas and his brother Isaac
are armed with waffled-cones full of
homemade food-processor icecream.
They love l'Agent Jean.
The drawings are high-impact colour fever dreams,
volumes signed by Alex A.
It's a sci-fi multiverse
populated with technicolour mammals and reptilians
with a variety of cybernetic cyborgisms.

Thomas comes to see me later at the dining table,
asks me if I want to learn more about Jean
and the "good guys" of the agency.
Henry is a nerdy lizard who's won 4 nobel prizes
but "ne parle pas anglais."
It's an archetypal story; Bond, made sillier.
Easy to believe this is the most fun reading around.
The kids have a book compiling all the characters and their metadata.
"But it's wrong! Colère first appeared in Tome 1, not Tome 4!"
Whiplash as we transition to playing tic-tac-toe.
Isaac demonstrates expertise in rigging the board,
but, I ask them, how inane is an unloseable game?

May 18th

It's evening, I am alone here.
No one else except, I realize, the cat.
I went out to the firepit and burned a letter,
watched the embers go out.
Back in the house,
I sit next to the cat
get to scratching, petting.
A low purr, and she moves into a better position for her.
Pads softly around me, I turn at the spine to follow.
Skull, neck, thorax, haunches. My hand runs over smoky fur.
She bends in, contorting to reach her sex with tongue
and licks herself avidly. Small body beats and
shudders until she suddenly stops, looks around.
The moment has passed.
I was merely some help, a privileged witness.

June 15th

Those movements of rivers overflowing
are the same as veins leaking.
A whisper in the poplar trees
I was tasked with trimming.
Saw off live branches, peel off the bark.
Notice inside the branch the artery bleeds red,
sickly sweet within white wood.
There will be no cure, I am healing myself.
I shed all regrets for every day in this life
that the sun rises and sets.
Nights spent in a tent to wake up
under the fury of Mars.
Ursa Major illuminating the barley field.
A harvest moon so bright I cast a shadow,
treading carefully so as not to trip,
seeking a key, the key that was stolen at birth,
So easy to get lost.

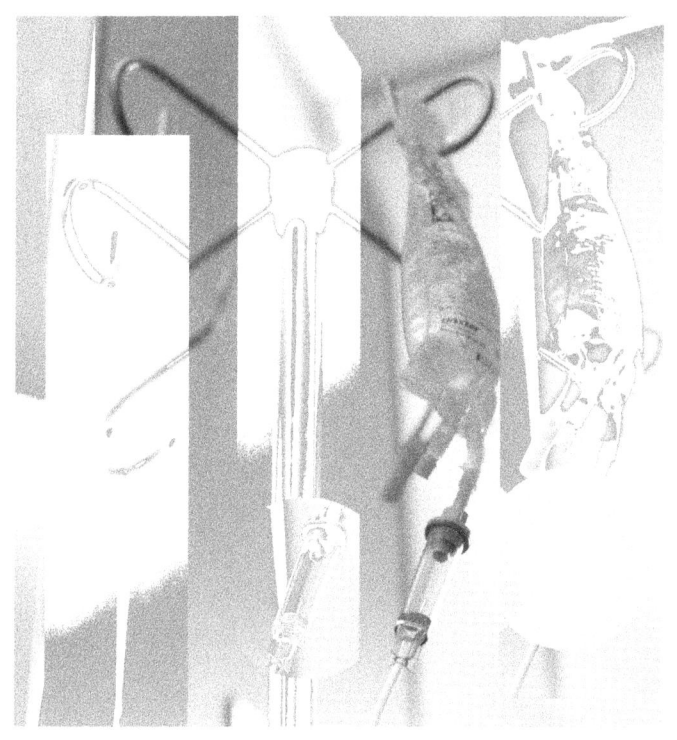

Surrender

Auto-Immune Manifesto

1. The transience of the body itself is holy.
2. Auto-immunity is self-defence, multifarious resistance, radical permeability, touchability.
3. Auto-immunity demands surrender, re-evaluation of what makes you human, what makes you you.
4. There is no such thing as health.
5. Auto-immunity shatters the telos upon shores of blood, treatment of symptoms agonizes the root cause.
6. Auto-immunity is not an illness, it is endowment with strength, power, knowledge.
7. Auto-immunity is self-knowledge, a map, responsibility.
8. Through auto-immunity, universal entanglements reverberate in felt sense.
9. Auto-immunity is not a curse, it is the wise wound within the body.
10. I would rather be sick and cunning than healthy and dull.
11. If I am sick, the land is sick.
12. Auto-immunity is the body in revolt against global poisoning.
13. Auto-immunity transcends identity.
14. Culture is auto-immune.
15. Auto-immunity diffracts the body's holistic context.
16. You can be auto-immune without conscious acceptance. Soon enough, your body will tell you.
17. Auto-immunity is a form of mourning; the body grieving worldly cruelty.
18. Auto-immunity is a call to listen.
19. Auto-immunity is inexorable change.
20. Auto-immunity is embodied heresy.
21. Auto-immunity is both constructive and destructive interference.
22. Auto-immunity is necessarily solitary, but you are not alone.

New Asceticism

WHAT DO I NEED?
  Enough food, a safe shelter, people with whom to share my life.
  Asceticism is about claiming the power to refuse.

The etymology has been traced to the 17th century,
from Medieval Latin asceticus,
from Ancient Greek ἀσκητικός (askētikós),
from ἀσκητής (askētḗs, "monk, hermit"),
from ἀσκέω (askéō, "I exercise").
There's the french word acèse, asceticism, abstention.

The god/dess of asceticism is Akeso,
daughter of Asclepius, the Physician of the gods.
Akeso is honest. Akeso is an alchemist. Akeso is temperance.
Sometimes harsh, sometimes gentle.
Always attuned to the needs of healing.
They do not heal so much as guide
the sick towards convalescence,
regeneration, re(in)storing their own capacity for recuperation.

From Ancient Greek Ἀκεσώ (Akesṓ).
In Portuguese, Galician, Italian, related to:
(transitive) to light, set alight, ignite, kindle
(transitive) to turn on (a device)
(transitive, figuratively) to fire up

So I read here a relation to training, practice,
an ongoing effort to deepen devotion and commitment.

The ascetic is traditionally a lone practitioner,
more closely related with the hermit
than the communal monastic (french: *cénobite*).
The ascetic need not preach, or attempt to convert others to their cause.

The definitions of asceticism I've found
commonly point towards either a moral practice or an artistic practice.
I am more aligned with ascesis as an art.
This is not a moral undertaking.
Rather, it is a response to global poisoning,
and a way to claim personal well-being,
individual action, pure negation.
Making space for something else.

My nascent asceticism acknowledges
that "the world" will not be saved,
that no saviour exists outside myself,
that supply chain collapse is ongoing,
that consumption wreaks havoc upon personal autonomy.
The practice involves learning to discern need from want,
sensing when want is an external imposition,
and refusing all that does not serve Life.

If, as Mircea Eliade suggests,
the sacred is defined spatially,
comes into being through delimitation,
exists as the exceptional place (Foucault's heterotopia),
then the Sacred is a standpoint to adopt,
a place from which to survey the wasteland,
and a devotee's habit to don as sheer refusal.

Refusal to engage with the profane,
refusal to inhabit the culture that continues to wreak havoc,
refusal to consume its commodities.
Rare is tuberculosis, yet how many still die consumptive?

Living a sacred life necessarily means acknowledging divinity;
not as god-almighty-on-high, merely as that-which-is.
For now, suffice to say divinity exists as an experience.
The metaphors for its facade are numerous.

Keep the practice joyful,
make room for physical pleasure,
sensuousness, salaciousness.
Refuse to imbibe the pornographer's easy meals.
Refuse the ready-to-think.
Refuse the pre-fabricated desires.
Abstain from cherry-picked realms of possibility.

Asceticism is the study of Life.
It is a syncretic approach,
meaning it takes what works from anywhere,
and refuses nonsense from anywhere.
In practice, the ascetic hones their sense of discernment,
their sensitivity, their bullshit detectors.

This is, ultimately, a game to play.
Inward, the search begins.
The search for that which is not spoken of.
But for whom is initiation an option in the first place?
And where, now, is the line between the speakable and the unspeakable?
Any wisdom gained will only be the wisdom of a dying civilization.
Pray to the old and new gods.
Worship in whatever way makes sense to you,
and do not expect your rites to make sense to your children.

Rites and ceremonies are potent tools.
From such movements arises gnosis,
deeply affecting practitioners and,
if devotion is sincere, changing the core of orientation to Life.
Ritual holds the power to transform one's own world,
and learn about the shared realities.
Ceremony alone, however, is hollow.
It is needfully directed by conscious control of the individual,
otherwise known as will, intent, attention, focus.
Without focus, ceremony is void of potency.

Some things are certain:
honestly performing established scripts leads to results,
and the results can profoundly alter experience.

Magic is a metaphor,
useful for making individual sense of patterns
that are too big to hold in the conscious mind.
It is an orientation device for mentation,
and useful for someone
who feels called to power for its own sake.
But why bother?

An ascetic approach acknowledges the ongoing process.
I inhabit the world of my own making,
while factors which I do not consciously hold in mind
continue to affect actions/decisions/options.

The theory is meaningless on its own.
Study for its own sake is navel-gazing.
Overloading intellect with big words
in the hope of spontaneously *getting it* leads nowhere,
not even disillusion. It is necessary to experiment, and to fail.
Whatever feels intuitive is a clue.
Whatever poses challenges but keeps interest is another.
There is much less to learn from other people than expected.
Auto-didactics are a key factor.
Desire is another. I want learning.
I want transformation.

Omnia mutantur

YOUR BODY IS LOOKING
for something for
itself for it's of concern
to feel here your body's situation
its (in)finitude.

Your body is trillions of microbes
billions of years in the making
destructive antibiotic abuse
microplastic, disintegrating commodities
alchemizing from fossil fragments,
deposits of Gaia's deep-time digestion
wreaking havoc upon microbiota
accumulated in the Pacific ocean
garbage patch; chlorella vulgaris
carefully cultivated freshwater
unicellular life, a fleeting grail
once touted as the solution
a solution?
to global food shortages
but really just another green powder;
like two and one-half billion grains of pollen
in a stainless-steel teaspoon,
gathered carefully over 240 hours
by the honeybee, marketed en-masse
as superfood; an elaborate
decentralized strategy
for population control.

My body is my grandmother Bluma,
I never met her,
her body displaced after Shoah
to a recently founded
military-colonial state
in 1951
My body is my father's faith,
alive against all odds in the year 5783
thousands of heretics burned,
drowned, and buried alive
in the name of one who was himself
martyred for heresy
the night flight of the sabbat
a mad crip prescribed Wellbutrin
in response to the complaint
"I am no longer able to read",
when really all I needed was to drop out
of the academy and find flourishing curiosity.
My body is twelve generations of colonizers
missionaries deforesting Gespe'gewa'gi
Family: Thirteen mouths
to feed under the watchful eye
of the parish priest,
the eldest raising the youth
while a burnt-out mother tends the father
Ailing near ending a life of physical toil
attempting to subdue the wild plot
25 acres offered to the white man
in exchange for his taxes, a contract
binding him to place, the alluring lie
that any human could own the earth
Five kilometres of prime salmon fishing
on the Gaspe's Restigouche river
controlled by the New York Elite
members of Brandy Brook fishing club.

I am my mother's
teenage longing
to get the fuck out of the backwoods
and travel the world;
the golden age of affordable gas prices
round-trip flights to Kathmandu
new age interfaith spirituality's disregard
for the complexities of syncretism
hailing the coming epoch
fifty years before seven planets
congress in Aquarius during the coronavirus'
first winter solstice;
A frenzied coked-out party
scene in Los Angeles,
fuelled by gore capitalism
black-market collaboration
with internationally operating
government institutions; British imperial
strategy for market control in China
through the trade in highly addictive drugs;
dimethyltriptamine vaporized
in my friend's downtown Montreal
loft during the height of a heatwave that killed
at least 7 people, a trip carried to the tune
of Chopin's
piano Nocturne No. 1 in B-flat Minor as rendered by
Vladimir Ashkenazy, an experience
of absolute certainty
that the universe is intelligent;
a gentle dialog with ghosts.

You are the tender blanket
of a lover's arms on a
pre-dawn morning
in the summer lockdown;
a twilit walk
along the Saint-Laurent
on stolen Mi'gmaq land
49 degrees north, past curfew,
the view:
stars reflected on
water, moist nostrils
frozen inhaling
stillness;
conversations with a stranger crossed along the footpath, his Saint Bernard kept off leash, in toe and quick to respond to a whistle, a man prone to flares of anger, yet always compassionate to the struggles of their food-desert of a village; a Quebecois father of four, labouring six months of the year to build housing infrastructure in the arctic circle for more workers to be flown up as machine operators in Agnico-Eagle's Nunavut gold mines;
open-pit rare-earth metal mining in
Baiyunebo leaching chemicals
the soil, acidifying
water bodies;
my macbook pro
purchased with student loan
debt 8 years ago,
on which I type this message; Sophie
Wilson, a trans woman
designing the ARM microprocessor 10
years before publicly transitioning;
Coccinelle taking synthetic oestrogen
in 1952 and working as a Paris
showgirl; Lynn Conway being
fired from IBM after stating
intent to medically transition,
barred from seeing her
children in 1969,
receiving an apology from the tech
giant 52 years later;

We are a tsunami;
elders in Fukushima
deciding to approach
the melting reactor
to spare the youth
radiation poisoning; the worship
of the written word; rising
and falling literate civilization;
academic overspecialization
and administrative data-entry
jobs; the stroke of a pen
ratifying the Paris climate accords;
Greenland refusing to join the agreement until
2021; rapidly melting ice sheets north of the 60th
parallel; 32 degrees celsius in Alaska mid-summer.

I am conceived in 1995, born in '96,
thinking
for sure I'll be dead by twenty-sixteen,
proven wrong;

I am a digital nomad, enjoying the banquet of international
festivals in Goa, Koh Phangan, Mazunte, and Istanbul;
a cybersecurity specialist working remotely to make sure
server infrastructure in Ukraine remains secure in a time
of active warfare; the displaced Oaxacan labourer farming
80 hours a week in California monocrop cultures to feed
the population of Edmonton strawberries in January; the
rise of industrial agriculture and the epidemic of food
allergies; made of the city's recycled sewage water; a
maple tree plantation; the goat-herd in the Mongolian
steppe producing cashmere for the global economic elite;
a desert wanderer fermenting ox milk in a hide bladder
slung around my waist on a day's march; Matzah baked the
day before Shabbat; tamari aged for years in American oak
barrels; evaporated ocean water leaving behind mineral
rich salts; the young Himalayan mountain range; a monk
lost in meditation, refusing to come down from the cave;
the Tesla Model T; greenwashing behind which hides
ongoing ecocide; lithium mines in Pilbara, Humboldt
County, Sonora, Harare, and James Bay; friendships formed
occupying Fairy Creek; the myth of progress; fires raging
at the library of Alexandria; Genesis; the Nag Hamadi
codex; walking through the Ishtar gate, contemplating
Etemenanki and dreaming of ecstatic ascent; Gobleki Tepe;
the blood of the earth; the genealogy of lactobacillus'
symbiosis with humanity; Jupiter's infinitesimal
gravitational pull upon the seas; Fat Man and Little Boy;
the project to colonize mars.

You are not a witch, not a druid, not a mystic, not a healer, not an expert, not trans, not a man, not a woman, not cis, not a unit, not a collective, not an esotericist, not a teacher, not buddhist, not christian, not jewish, not muslim, not indigenous, not an initiate, not an inventor, not a prophet, not god, not an anarchist, not a liberal, not conservative, not a radical, not a marxist, not a leftist, not right-wing, not a maoist, not a leninist, not a foucauldian, not a deleuzian, not sick, not healthy, not complete, not human, not docile, not domestic, not feral, not wild, not calm, not angry, not vociferous, not a pagan, not sumerian, not babylonian, not a sorcerer, not a priest/ess, not a worker, not a nietzschean, not an egoist, not a communist, not a libertarian, not committed, not a thief.

We are cholera; measles landing on turtle island in 1492;
the cross erected at Gaspe point in 1534; forest fires
turning the sky red over the Salish Sea in 2020; the amnesiac
Kid wandering Bellona, outside of time;
a Kalashnikov rifle handed to a child;
ritualized violence and desacralized warfare;
human savagery and the tenderness of wolves.

My body is Akeso tending to the fever dreams of the
incubatio at Epidaurus; corporate state surveillance; the
Googleplex; a datacenter air-conditioned year-round to 21
degrees celsius; the burnt-out nihilistic activist
watching news feeds cycle endlessly through nonsense; a
brutal end to the holocene climactic optimum; drought,
famine, flood; the return of chaos; a quiet seed of hope.

You are our friend's embrace
welcoming us home after a 14 hour red-eye;
a look of despair in your roommate's eyes,
coming back from the slaughter
a hundred chickens our community bought, fed, and raised
to have food for winter;
those fowls' bones dissolving in a marrow-rich broth;
catharsis; the remembering of limitless interconnectivity;
an autonomous healer, having chosen to stop taking meds,
and surviving; regenerative decay;
society without states;
the remembrance of life looking nothing like this;
a bacterium alive in the heart of a volcano;
acceptance of what is;
an initiatrix of revolution, discovering new Devi;
the fall of patriarchy;
the laughter of generations to come;

We are simple fireside conversation concerned only with local affairs;
an expedition to a perennial berry patch in early autumn;
plantain leaf poultice applied to mosquito bites;
the dissolution of animosity upon realization of essential unity;
neighbours greeted warmly;
a child mocked by the innocent curiosity of their peers,
scarred disfigured face made unforgettable by chance;
a dancer following only the rhythms of breath;
collective nervous system co-regulation;
a quiet city without combustion engines;
future old growth; custodian to a food forest;
the circle around which humans sit to resolve their problems;
common horsetail, labelled invasive, full of medicine;
new folklore, found in searching; a story of fabulous tides;
a child contemplating the southern fish
from a bed of yarrow stalks on a moonless night;
tears of mourning;
blissful release; eternally young;
resulting of decisions made long before our birth;

A Birthday Poem
2022-02-21

How do I learn to not speak?
    Always speaking the future changes it,
    makes it slip away.

    Speak sparingly if at all
    Sharpen thought to an arrowhead
    What naïveté to rush
    the tree in its bearing fruit

    Je réalise quelque chose
    c'est tout simple
    Je refuse de risquer
    ma vie, ma santé
    Pour gagner des miettes.

    Mais pourtant j'ai une trajectoire
    L'idée d'origine
    Celle pour laquelle
    je quittai la ville
    L'exploration/L'apprentissage
    de cette forêt.

    Connaître l'arbre requiert
    dormir sous ses frondes
    amourachée parmi les bourgeons
    Danser dans les vergers
    Connaître l'arbre demande
    des rêves remplis de sucreries

Si ce n'est un poème
du moins ce sera une histoire.
C'est un jour de retour et d'arrivée
Si cette journée m'apporte mélancolie
accompagnant les voeux
cela doit être signe que l'hiver tire à sa fin
Dernier quart de lune pour un début, retour
autour de ce soleil salvateur

Absurd hilarious horror we know
it's about not knowing until it's
already happened
So I laugh
at my silly sense of self-aggrandizement

The crux of my problems lately is that I feel useless
So, find a way to be useful

Consciente, je rêve
d'affectivité expérimentale
d'épaves, où jouir d'entregens
d'énergie, de dynamisme chaotique
Je répercute toutes les entraves
qui me traversent
et le défi, c'est
simplement de remarquer
les clôtures

Attention, ce qui fut commun fut saisit
Feu, y mettre feu
Tout braquer, détruire ce qui m'étrangle
ce qui me noue, la gorge
sèche, asséché, vide
de sens à boire sans cesse
ces eaux ce chlore
pour s'empoisonner
consciemment
je dois guérir.

C'est qu'à 20 ans
je me suis réveillée
J'ai réalisé que je suis
vivante, encore vivante.
C'est qu'à 25 ans j'ai découvert
mon ignorance, j'ai apprivoisé mon deuil.
C'est qu'aujourd'hui, la fatigue me lorgne
et je n'y peux toujours rien.

Alors j'imagine le printemps
J'imagine un monde créé collectivement
qui n'a rien à foutre
de la droite et la gauche

J'imagine des sentiers en terre battue
sur lesquels ne roulent aucune ferraille

J'imagine une vie parsemée de déplacements
s'effectuant uniquement à pied.

J'imagine la santé pour toustes

J'imagine une humanité
fortement réduite
Réapprivoisant cette terre
la seule que nous ayons

J'imagine la fin du cauchemar industriel.

Je m'imagine que la mort est nécessaire à la naissance
tout comme la pause est nécessaire à l'acte.

J'imagine volontiers un éden devenu désert
avec les fausses promesses de ces textes
millénaires enfin mises à nues.

Je rêve de défaire tout
ce que mes ancêtres blancs,
gaspésiens depuis 300 ans,
ont commis dans l'ignorance et la hâte

Je rêve de faire des choix
qui feront l'honneur et non la honte
de mes descendantes.

Si c'est vrai qu'il faut penser
pour sept générations
Je me demande bien ce qu'imaginaient
les colons dont je naquis
celleux qui avaient
30 arpents et plus;
considéraient-iels
le vol, le meurtre?

Et moi, en ai-je vraiment conscience?

J'imagine ce qui viendra après
Puis je me souviens qu'une définition possible de l'anarchie, c'est:
"sans début ni fin"

Alors il n'y aurait que maintenant
Ici; où l'éternel pénètre le temporel
Parmi nous.
Et si la mélancolie m'accompagne
en ce jour, ce n'est pas à défaut
de rêves, de joie. Si la tristesse
est présente, c'est qu'elle l'est
toujours, vivant en temps de deuil.

Alors j'imagine le soleil
et les amix
et les abeilles
et je me dis que chaque moment
vécu pleinement
est en soi une forme révolutionnaire
Et chaque rêve raconté
me rapproche du monde désiré
de l'autre côté de cette folie collective
que les dormeurs ne remarquent même pas.

All Things Change

THIS 25TH YEAR OF my life marks a shift.
  As all rites of passage, I had to shed any notions of knowing
  who, where, when, and why I was.
  As all thresholds, the other side was invisible from the entryway,
  unknown and unknowable to me.

  The morass of digital communication weighs heavy,
  and isolation is not aided by over-engagement.
  I discern conflicting impulses within myself,
  doubts and trust coexisting, and feel on the verge of birth.
  Perhaps this is because I will soon turn 26.
  Perhaps this is because the past year has held
  inexpressable lows and vertiginous highs.

  I had ceased all medical supervision,
  believing then, as i do now,
  that I am better equipped to heal myself
  than any other doctor.

  Hubris was my downfall,
  as were a series of mistakes
  stemming from hurried action
  chasmic gaps in my own knowledge.

  The refusal to take my pills had the effect
  of revealing symptoms that had lain dormant for a decade.
  I precipitated this, stepping wildly through a thick fog
  on the frozen banks of the river sainte-anne, praying,
  hoping that health would occur spontaneously.

Now, where I then had only fear and longing,
I now have words to describe that particular crisis of healing.
An inapt diet was the catalyst for toxemia
and the emergence of dysbiosis,
or, the sheer destruction of the microbiome
whch protects and regulates my organism.

I was vulnerable, my gut homeostasis was fragile
from 20 years of regular subjection to antiobiotics and other poisons.
My years of binge drinking taught me,
eventually, the value of abstention,
but not how to go about caring for a body
taxed heavily by the drugs of modern life.

From the moment I started drinking, I abused my liver.
From the day I got on Revolade, I imposed undue stress on my liver.
It's where I am now holding tension still.
Right where the diaphragm meets the top of the liver.

So a year ago, I was alone with my symptoms.
I decided then the drug I'd been prescribed
and taking since 2015 would still be of use.
A new doctor took the place of the old.
This specialist I've never met,
and whose voice I only ever hear in 10 minute increments,
mobilized the machine of pharmacy.
The wait for renewal, mere weeks, was too long.
Blood tests indicated a need for emergency treatments.
So, under the needle and the crystalline bag I went.
I partook in the logistical ritual of medicine once more.
The top floor of the CISSS de la Haute-Gaspésie
welcomes me onto the colonized land of Gespe'gewa'gi.
Sterile, this new waiting room.
I wait patiently until Marie calls me to her,
and I walk to treatment, my bright blue-slippered feet
follow her to the hall of recliners.

I've learned compassion from the plasma of strangers.
The 21st century corruption of the gift relationship
has joined us locally, mixed our waters.
Birth circumstances on this artificially fractured continent
place us on either side of a free trade agreement.
My doctor's signature on the prescription
reaches across time and binds me to the donors
whose act expedites my temporary cure.
The thousands become my bio-spiritual ancestors
and theirs are lessons to heed in the blood.
How am I to understand transfusion?
It's a slow remembering, a reconstruction.
Drop by crystal drop the infusion is vetted, approved, absorbed.
The memory is wholly mine, but the blood is legion.
I won't pretend to understand all the mechanisms at work
pharmacokinetics and the like.
Medicine has its explanations for what I've undergone;
This pamphlet is my own interpretation.

I'm struggling to make sense
of what those 72 hours post-IVIG mark in my life.
I had just turned 25. I was looking for answers,
having not yet learned that, at best,
I can merely refine my questions.

At the time, it felt like something profound ought to come from agony.
But perhaps it is the banality, the ultimate meaninglessness of side-effects
that is revealed here. What right have I to claim some importance,
to ascribe meaning to the everyday? Remember this: we all suffer.

The meaning is not in the suffering itself.
    How could I possibly justify painkillers if it were?
    Is sense experience inherently meaningful?
Is anaesthesia, then, a poison, chilling the soul
    as well as the body?
Ought I have let the migraine run its course
    without those little tylenol pills?
What experience or insight did I deprive myself of
    by choosing to minimize pain?
Is this line of questioning merely playing
    into a masochist hero's narrative?
Or a fantasy of the tortured mystic?
Another question in progress:
How do the pharmaco-kinetics of intravenous blood products
affect bio-spiritually intra-acting bodies?
Simple: I do not know.

In the midst of pandemic,
I shed many of my preconceived notions
I had long held about my own reality.
I was (and am) giving serious consideration
to the aspects of my experience
that I could not fit into a materialist framework.

I dove, alone, ever deeper into myself,
away from as much of the noise as I could,
and found faith in the existence of divinity on earth.

I found that even as I critically examine
the claims of charlatans
and continue to reject their postural pretences,
their false certainties, their easy assurances,
there is an intangible, indefinite, inner resonance
to the notion that this human body
is a direct conduit for my experience of god.

I know now that healing is a series of definite mechanisms
harnessing the body's innate capacity for adaptation.
My path is aligned with the middle way, the way of the heart.
I am neither shunning my embodied state,
nor am I attached to it as a stable, unshifting identity.
Without striving towards any spiritual goal,
I remain aware of the continual tension between edifice and dissolution.

I practice in order to neither hold on to my biographical history
as the sole source of my identity, nor relinquish
the potential for transformation that inheres
to the condition of being alive as a human being.

Jouissance is an aspect of the art of getting lost.
Creative forgetfulness is part of the way.
Internal alchemy is the process of consciously rearranging one's inner be-
    ing.

I am not enlightened, nor is it true that I know nothing at all.
I am slowly knowing myself, and I know what I've learned,
what I've experienced. I know some of what I do not know.
I am not merely an empty vessel for divinity,
but a collaborator with the universal forces.
Being me is a worthwhile endeavour in and of itself,
and so is noting the patterns that have calcified
over the course of my life so far.

The river thaws, its flows inexorable.
I practice lovingkindness for the land itself,
the boulders in Rivière-Du-Loup's Parc Des Chutes, the moss.
May they be at peace, free from suffering.
Hollow human words for a stone,
yet the resonance from the heart center is true, real.

What does the land need?
Time, which it has.
Love, presence, acknowledgement.
The dirt is not alone, I am here.
We are here, those of us who are awake
with compassion for the web of life.

AUTO-IMMUNE HERESY

Hold the bodies close together
and find they resolve into
dissolution, disillusion. One
flesh precludes not another.
One voice does not make a chorus.

Listen to the silence of the hum-
drum daily affairs, and find
cracks through which to slip
in which to get lost. Only
with loss does the finding
have meaning. Only after does
before have value. Not a comparison
to draw between discrete units
but an exponential resonance
when the cycle is acknowledged
in its full ongoing dream.

Smaller, still
2022-08-22

So many options &
    some are true but
    few and far between
    come from the honest calling

    Ready to do not doing
    Practice insight
    Clear some shadows
    Learn thyself

    Maybe just
    do nothing
    over
    and over
    and over
    until the moment
    of truth

    Dynamism gives takes
    push pull

    Language weighs heavy
    words create mere illusion

    And so I am an illusionist
    seeking to find release
    from the bondage of my silver tongue.

On July 8th , 2022, I journaled:
"where's that feeling of enoughness?"
Satiety needs not just food.
It asks intimacy, touch, connection.
I believe in love and creation.
Life is infinite imagination.
Culture is malleable clay.
Remember pain is part of the work.
An integral piece of healing is hurt.
The wise wounds are the teachers.

At the end // À Suivre

A long winding path, tremulously lit.
Traveler, there is no road.

I am crossing time
each of my selves
conceived otherwise
leap through one another in memory.

The road is made as you go
But tell me more about this path.
It is ever present, shifting
Not to accommodate,
Though it remains navigable.
Divergences cease to exist
Once a decision has been made
The path is only travelled once
Though it may come back around.
Each day along the path brings new learning
The feeling of the path changes
Come now, you're already on your way
The path is shared by all, and differs for each.

As of writing, it is January 2024.

I have been in remission for two years.
My last dose of IVIG was Feb 2021.
I haven't set foot in a hospital since December 2021.

I stopped taking my platelet boosters,
self-supervised, without any Doctor's orders.
I haven't taken any pharmaceutical medicine since March 2022.
The seeds of my practice are all present in this book, if you look for them.

I have given myself to the art of nourishing life.

I am changing.
The process will never be complete,
because it is not something with an end goal.
I have befriended my body.
I sing, and dance, and pray.

The story laid out in the preceding pages is only a fraction of reality.
Forgive me, that I could not be more thorough.
This edition of the book arose out of a need to publish quickly,
an irresistible urge to finish.
As such, I take full responsibility for any errors, typos, repetition,
or other mistakes that would have been easily resolved
by working with more time,
but the text asked to see the light of day.

This remains but a fragment,
there is so much more to life.

I am publishing this book to open a dialogue.
In honour of all those who've come before
and all those who've yet to arrive.

Selected Bibliography

Books:

Bellamie, Dodie. When The Sick Rule The World.
Crary, Jonathan. 24/7: Late Capitalism and the Ends of Sleep.
Foucault, Michel. Surveiller et punir: naissance de la prison.
Grey and Dimech, The Brazen Vessel, Scarlet Imprint.
Hiromu Awaraka, Fullmetal Alchemist.
Kafer, Alison. Feminist, Queer, Crip.
Preciado, Paul B., TESTO YONQUI
SUSAN SONTAG, ON PHOTOGRAPHY.
Stacy Alaimo, Bodily Natures.
Sozialistisches Patientenkollektiv, Turn Illness into a Weapon: For Agitation.

Articles and Web

ABC News. 'Why Thousands of Low-Income Americans "Donate" Their Blood Plasma'. ABC News_, 14 Jan. 2017, https://abcnews.go.com/US/thousands-low-income-americans-donate-blood-plasma-profit/story?id=44710257. Accessed 28 Oct. 2018.
Blood Plasma Donation Tips. *How Much Do You Get Paid to Donate Plasma?*. Dec. 2016, http://www.plasmadonating.net/2013/03/how-much-do-you-get-paid-to-donate.html. Accessed 25 Nov. 2018.
CSL Behring. PRODUCT MONOGRAPH Privigen® Immunoglobulin Intravenous (Human) 10 % Solution for Infusion. 2019.

CSL Plasma. *Testing and Processing Plasma*. https://www.cslplasma.com/about-csl-plasma/testing-and-processing-plasma. Accessed 20 Feb. 2021

CSL Plasma. Make Cash, Save Lives - Start Donating at CSL Plasma Today!, https://www.youtube.com/watch?v=DfLi3QBuUWU. Accessed 28 Feb. 2020.

Jolles, S., et al. 'Clinical Uses of Intravenous Immunoglobulin'. Clinical and Experimental Immunology, vol. 142, no. 1, Oct. 2005, pp. 1. PubMed Central, doi:10.1111/j.1365-2249.2005.02834.x.,

Ludwin, Steven, and S. Ryan Greysen. 'Use of Smartphones and Mobile Devices in Hospitalized Patients: Untapped Opportunities for Inpatient Engagement'. Journal of Hospital Medicine, vol. 10, no. 7, Apr. 2015, pp. 459–61. doi:10.1002/jhm.2365.

Perez, Elena E., et al. 'Update on the Use of Immunoglobulin in Human Disease: A Review of Evidence'. Journal of Allergy and Clinical Immunology, vol. 139, no. 3, Mar. 2017, pp. S1–46. Crossref, doi:10.1016/j.jaci.2016.09.023.

Slonim, Robert, et al. 'The Market for Blood'. Journal of Economic Perspectives. vol. 28, no. 2, May 2014, pp. 177–96. www.aeaweb.org, doi: 10.1257/jep.28.2.177.

Scantibodies Biologics. 'Donate Plasma, Help Save Lives and Get Cash! Its Very Easy!' _Scantibodies Biologics, http://www.scantibodiesbiologics.com. Accessed 28 Oct. 2018. In the midst of pandemic, the website shows the following notice: "Dear Donors, Due to COVID-19 impact, SBI Plasma Center is regrettably forced to suspend operations until the pandemic is over. We are thankful for all your plasma donations and we hope to be able to welcome you back soon to continue saving lives together." Accessed 14 March 2022.

Weston, Kath. 'Lifeblood, Liquidity, and Cash Transfusions: Beyond Metaphor in the Cultural Study of Finance'. Journal of the Royal Anthropological Institute, vol. 19, May 2013, pp. 537. Crossref, doi:10.1111/1467-9655.12014

About Laure

I am on a pilgrimage
back to my own body.

My current research is engaged in
mapping my homunculus, and learning yangsheng, which translates literally as "the art of nourishing life."

養生
*yang-
sheng*

A generous community of patrons supports my work
via my website's membership.
To keep up with the ongoing journey
and show your support, you can visit
<u>www.laure.love</u>
and you can email:
contact@laure.love

Thank you for everything.

www.ingramcontent.com/pod-product-compliance
Lightning Source LLC
Chambersburg PA
CBHW040222040426
42333CB00050B/3293